FRENCH PARADOX

and Beyond

Living Longer With Wine and the Mediterranean Lifestyle

By

LEWIS PERDUE

With An Introduction and Chapters by:

KEITH MARTON, M.D., F.A.C.P.

Chairman, Department of Medicine, California Pacific Medical Center

Associate Clinical Professor, University of California, San Francisco Medical School

and

WELLS SHOEMAKER, M.D., F.A.A.P.

Practicing Pediatrician

Founder, Intensive Care Nursery, Watsonville Hospital

Renaissance Publishing

Sonoma, California

NOTICE

This book is intended as a reference volume only, not as a substitute for medical advice which should come from your physician. If you suspect that you have a medical problem or a problem with alcohol, we suggest that you contact your physician immediately.

The information here is intended to help you make informed decisions on diet, lifestyle and alcohol consumption but cannot be considered a substitute for proper medical advice, treatment and supervision.

Published by
Renaissance Publishing,
867 W. Napa St., Sonoma, CA 95476

Copyright © 1992 by Renaissance Publishing
All rights reserved. No part of this publication may be reproduced or transmitted in any form or by any means, electronic or mechanical including photocopying, recording or any other information storage or retrieval system without the written permission of the publisher.

Distributed to the book trade by Publishers Group West, Emeryville, CA.

Printed in the United States of America on acid-free, recycled paper.

Book design by Lisa Burnette

CONTENTS

PART I
The Facts on Wine, Food and Health

Chapter One 2

French Paradox? No, No: It's An American Paradox

We're the ones spending billions on health care and fitness clubs. So why are the French blowing Gauloise smoke in our faces and outliving us to boot?

Chapter Two 15

Leading a Longer, Disease-Free Life

This book promises to help you decrease your chances of getting a heart attack, live a healthier life without deprivation, and make your own independent decisions about the health studies reported in the press.

Sidebar One 20

What is Alcohol, Anyway?

It's nearly impossible to avoid in food or nature.

Chapter Three 24

What's All the Fuss About?

Why are people suddenly so interested in wine and health?

Sidebar Two 33

What's a Drink?

Defining how much is a drink.

Chapter Four 34

What's Wrong With Intervention? Plenty!

Treatments once you have a heart attack have lots of problems: you could die before getting to a hospital; it's expensive, painful and doesn't always work.

Chapter Five 38

Aging Gracefully With Wine

Moderate alcohol consumption is a strong indicator of seniors who stay active and healthy as they grow older.

Sidebar Three 41

Beware of "Popular" Alcohol Advice

Much of what you read is based on outdated, distorted or intentionally biased data.

Chapter Six 44

Is It The Wine or the Food? Yes...And No

Food is an important factor in staying healthy, but the greatest body of scientific data points to moderate alcohol consumption as one of the most important factors in living longer.

Sidebar Four 53

Wine and Diabetes

Diabetics need not avoid alcohol, but must choose their beverage carefully and with their doctor's advice

Sidebar Five 55

Wine and Gout

Gout is not caused by alcohol consumption, but can be aggravated by heavy drinking and abuse.

Chapter Nineteen 147

Wine, Pregnancy and Fetal Alcohol Syndrome

The problem is abuse, not moderate consumption. What are the real facts and why have some "advocacy" groups tried to frighten women with misinformation? To keep them barefoot and pregnant?

Chapter Twenty 161

Breastfeeding and Alcohol

Mothers need not worry about the moderate glass of vino.

Chapter Twenty-One 164

Keeping Youth From Abusing Alcohol

"Just say no," doesn't work with sex, drugs, rock and roll or alcohol.

Sidebar Eleven 170

One Pediatrician's Observations on Preventing Youth Alcohol Abuse

Experience with the growing-up pains of hundreds of children offers some perspective.

PART III
The Science of Wine and Health

Chapter Twenty-Two 174

Avoiding Junk Science: How to Make Your Own Decisions

In an age of "factlets" and sound bites, a lot of people with hidden agendas are trying to distort science for their own goals. How do you separate the gems from the junk?

Sidebar Twelve 183

"Proving" a Scientific Impossibility

How scientists once used junk science to "prove" that education made women less fertile.

Chapter Twenty-Three 184

Why Do Heart Attacks Happen?

It's more than just a plumbing problem for the medical Roto-Rooters

Chapter Twenty-Four 190

Cholesterol & Fats: Jekyll and Hyde Characters

We can't live without them, but they can be the death of us all.

Chapter Twenty-Five 202

Why Do Coronary Arteries Clog Up?

Diet, stress and heredity all play a role.

Sidebar Thirteen 211

Strokes of Misfortune

How alcohol may prevent some cerebrovascular disease or put you at risk.

PART IV
The Cookbook

Eat Easy, Healthy & Delicious 242

Thirty-nine brand-new recipes to get you started on eating in the Mediterranean style.

Part V
About The Authors

Doctors, Scientists and a Journalist 266

Just who are the people behind this book? What are their qualifications and biases?

Introduction

Dr. Keith Marton, M.D.
Chairman, Department of Medicine, California Pacific Medical Center
Associate Clinical Professor, University of California, San Francisco Medical School

The French Paradox

Despite its growing technologic orientation, medicine still deals primarily in the collection, interpretation and transmission of information. Practitioners of internal medicine, such as myself, are especially concerned with this process.

While many people think of doctors as spending most of their time diagnosing and treating illness, I think of physicians as teachers. Why is that? Because so much of what happens with respect to a person's health is under that person's control and can therefore be taught. No, we can not control our heredity nor can we account for simple bad luck.

However, lifestyle decisions, which account for a very high proportion of health-related issues, are under our control. Moreover, how we deal with illness (i.e. how we live with disability and discomfort, how we choose to take medications and whether or not we opt for one treatment or another) are also under our control. In these areas, the physician can simply advise, not dictate.

In my own experience, most people prefer to see their physicians function as counselors, providing the information that allow them to make their own informed decisions. The clearer the information, the clearer the choices; the clearer the potential outcomes, the more prepared each person is to make such informed decisions.

There are times in medicine where choices are very clear: few of us would refuse to have our broken arm placed in a cast; we all agree to take antibiotics for pneumonia. Most decisions, however, are not so cut and dried: the options are many and the uncertainty is great. The person who has had a heart attack can opt to take medication (from which there are many to choose), have a balloon dilatation of their coronary arteries, or undergo coronary bypass surgery.

Each approach has its own set of risks, costs and benefits . The uncertainty comes from the observation that few things in life (particularly approaches to health care) are proven and etched in stone. What was good for us 20 years ago may be anathema now, simply because of the changing winds of scientific research.

This is no more true than in the area of lifestyle choices. In the last 40 years, our attitudes as a society have changed radically when it comes to issues such as diet, exercise and early detection of disease. As the reader will see in the following chapters, there is a great deal of debate about many aspects of alcohol use. While the negative consequences of alcohol abuse are clear, the balance of risks and benefits for more moderate use remains debatable in many circles. Even in the area of the cardio-protective effects of alcohol, where the research is extraordinarily robust and convincing, one could argue that the cardio-protective effect of alcohol is not strictly "proven". That is, no one has ever done a randomized, controlled trial in which half of the people receive alcohol and half do not. It is unlikely that such a study will ever be done, given our societal penchant for freedom of personal choice, and given our societal concern for the ethics of prescribing a potentially addicting substance. If this is so, then each of us is going to have to make an individual decision about whether or not we choose to drink, since the medical evidence will never be strictly one-sided.

The other thing that medical data does not always take into account is quality of life. When it comes to the enjoyment of a glass of wine, many of us believe that quality of life considerations are paramount. Only the individual can know how to truly value the enjoyment that comes from a nice meal with friends or loved ones. No study can tell us what this really means.

Studies that evaluate the role of alcohol in breast cancer and fetal development raise other very personal issues: how do we evaluate potential risks and compare them with very personal benefits? No physician or policy maker can truly dictate what is right. It remains the privilege of the individual to make such difficult decisions. Those of us who believe in the intelligence of the American adult believe books such as this are an important addition: they do not tell the person how to behave. Rather, they provide information with which reasoned choices can be made.

In the meantime, let me salute each reader of this book with what should be the rallying cry of all physicians: To Your Health!

Keith Marton, M.D.

San Francisco

July, 1992

Preface

This book is designed to present an accurate and balanced picture of wine, alcohol, the Mediterranean lifestyle, and how you can put it to work in your own life to cut your risk of heart attacks and live a longer, more enjoyable life.

As the principal author, I searched for all the credible, scientifically sound material, good or bad, and put it in here. I restricted the definition of "credible, scientifically sound" to medical and scientific journals (such as *the New England Journal of Medicine, The Lancet, Cardiology, The Journal of the American Medical Association*) where the materials are rigorously examined and peer-reviewed by true scientists.

There is a large body of pseudoscientific materials which have been ignored because of the lack of scientific standards, the presence of a political agenda, the lack of credible scientific credentials by the authors (a Ph.D. in sociology is rarely able to make valid scientific conclusions in medicine or biochemistry) and because I, like most people, feel a lot more comfortable putting my health in the hands of an M.D. instead of the hands of a Ph.D. in social work.

After writing the manuscript, all of the chapters were reviewed by collaborators Drs. Marton and Shoemaker. In addition, a number of the other chapters -- including those dealing with alcohol and cardiac health -- were reviewed for accuracy by Dr. Curtis Ellison.

This book is designed for each chapter to stand on its own; understanding a given chapter does not mean having to read all the previous chapters. For this reason, there is a small amount of redundancy in a few of the chapters, but I have tried to keep that at a minimum.

To your health!

Lewis Perdue

July, 1992

Acknowledgments

My deepest thanks go to:

- Keith Marton, M.D., who provided me with copies of his medical and scientific research compiled over the past ten years and wrote the introduction to this edition.
- Wells Shoemaker, M.D., who wrote a number of original chapters for this book and whose offbeat sense of humor made me laugh in the middle of all the grinding work that it took to write this.
- Keith, Wells and Curtis Ellison, M.D., for their reviews of the manuscript and their innumerable suggestions for changes (all of which were made).
- Mary Evelyn Arnold who edited the book in record time and made a vital contribution to the manuscript's readability.
- Experienced cooks Dorothy Mills of Orinda, Calif., and Adam Gold of Seattle, Wash. for kitchen testing all of the book recipes and making valuable changes which improved the lot.
- My wife, Megan, who has now endured 14 books without killing or leaving me. None of my books, nor any other accomplishment would have been possible without her and the sacrifices she has made.

Lewis Perdue

July 1992

ONE

The *American* Paradox!

The French outlive Americans by about two and a half years (76.5 versus 74) and suffer 40 percent fewer heart attacks despite the fact that Gauloise smoking is a national pastime, their diet swims in a torrent of fat and the average Gaul speaks the language of Nautilus, StairStepper and aerobics about as well as English (or any other barbarian tongue). Despite all our billions spent on health care, and the sweat and the self denial, and the bland health food diets, we still die younger. And some would say that at the end of this journey, we didn't enjoy the scenery nearly as much as the average French peasant.

Health is on the plate and in the glass; it's just politically incorrect to recognize those facts.

This situation has been dubbed "The French Paradox" and was made famous in November, 1991, when CBS's Morley Safer explored the matter on an episode of *60 Minutes.*

In reality, the whole bubbling cauldron of contradictions should be labeled "The American Paradox" because we have, at our everyday convenience, all of the means to match and surpass the French levels of *joie de vivre* and health success. But we refuse to recognize or do anything about them, partly because the answers seem too simple, partly because our health philosophy focuses on intervention rather than prevention and partly because of hysterical opposition to alcohol consumption in any quantity at all. For the reality is that health is on the plate and in the glass; it's just politically incorrect to recognize those facts.

According to Dr. R. Curtis Ellison, M.D., chief of preventive medicine and epidemiology and professor at Boston University School of Medicine, the French secret boils down to wine, food and lifestyle.

The French, Dr. Ellison says:

- Are regular consumers of moderate amounts of alcohol, especially red wine, primarily with meals,
- Eat more fresh fruit and vegetables,
- Take longer to eat meals and snack less,
- Eat less red meat,
- Eat more cheese, less whole milk and
- Use more olive oil and less lard or butter.

Of all these factors, Dr. Ellison said the link with moderate and regular consumption of wine with meals is the strongest and most scientifically proven.

In fact, Dr. Ellison's list is an exhortation for a "back to the future" approach to dietary health which embraces more traditional, healthier cuisines (and their associated moderate wine consumption). We shouldn't rely on processed "techno-foods" like Simplesse, Nutrasweet, MacLean Burgers and "Lite" foods which manufacturers have manipulated beyond recognition in order to make them "healthier."

Greg Drescher, a director of the Massachusetts-based Oldways Preservation and Exchange Trust (which is dedicated to preserving traditional cuisines), draws an analogy between techno-foods and methadone: "We don't know where we're going with that approach; the cure may be worse than the disease," he said. "Techno-food could prove dangerous." By contrast, he says traditional cuisines are tried and true sources of health.

One of the first San Francisco Bay Area restaurants to put the traditional ways into practice was Chez Panisse which, for more than 20 years, has emphasized fresh, natural and organic ingredients -- but all without throwing the health aspects in the diner's face.

"I don't want to interfere with people," says owner and chef Alice Waters, "telling them, 'you are eating politically correct biologically wholesome food.' It gets tedious."

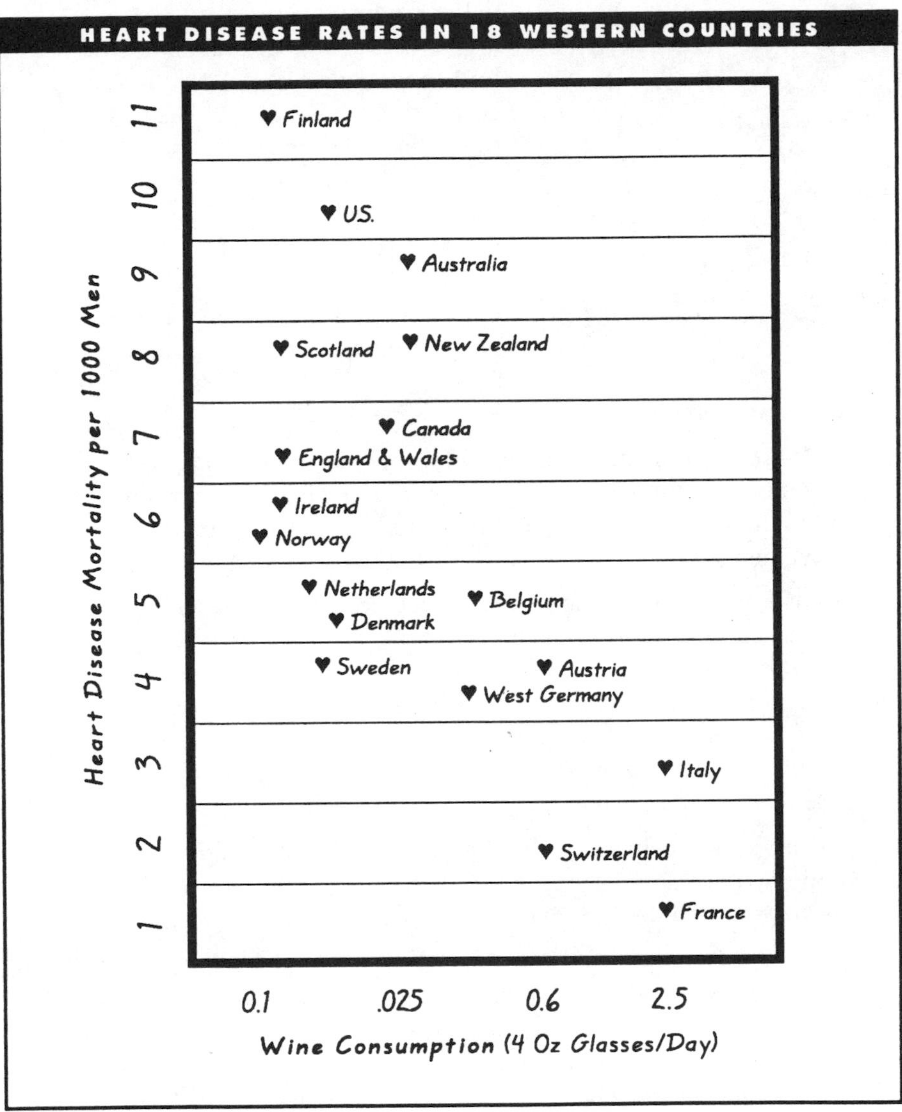
HEART DISEASE RATES IN 18 WESTERN COUNTRIES
Heart Disease Mortality per 1000 Men
11
10
9
8
7
6
5
4
3
2
1
Finland
US.
Australia
Scotland
New Zealand
Canada
England & Wales
Ireland
Norway
Netherlands
Belgium
Denmark
Sweden
Austria
West Germany
Italy
Switzerland
France
0.1
.025
0.6
2.5
Wine Consumption (4 Oz Glasses/Day)

Source: St. Leger. The Lancet. 1979

Moderate drinkers have a significantly lower death rate (usually 20 to 40 percent less)* from all causes *than abstainers and even lower rates than heavy drinkers.

But traditional cuisines are coming under commercial pressure not only in fast/frozen/processed/manufactured/techno-food America, but in the very cradle of healthy cuisine -- France and the Mediterranean. The British magazine, *New Scientist*, reports that a European food industry research firm, Leatherhead Food Research Association, is offering for sale an expensive study that identifies opportunities for selling processed foods to consumers in the Mediterranean countries.

"There is considerable potential for manufactured food products in Italy, Spain, Portugal and Greece," said a Leatherhead news release. "And there is already a definite trend towards processed and convenience foods at the expense of the fresh sector."

It is ironic then that the first broadside fired in defense of traditional French cuisine came from the big guns of American television, *60 Minutes*, and that the concept would be kept alive by the American wine industry which is mounting a massive publicity campaign to promote the health benefits of wine and French/Mediterranean food culture. Americans in defense of French culture? *Mon Dieu!* The American paradox continues.

During that segment on *60 Minutes*, Dr. Serge Renaud, M.D., head of the Lyon center of INSERM (the French equivalent of our National Institutes of Health) said, "It's well documented that a moderate intake of alcohol prevents coronary heart disease by as much as 50 percent."

Dr. Renaud's assertion is backed by scores of university and hospital studies, conducted at places like Harvard and Cornell, and published in such respected publications as the *Journal of the American Medical Association*, *The American Journal of Cardiology* and the leading British medical journal, *Lancet*. Some of the studies are as recent as 1992 and others date back to the mid-1920s.

But what is moderate? According to Dr. Keith Marton, M.D., chairman of the Department of Medicine at the California Pacific Medical Center and a professor at the University of California, San Francisco Medical School, "moderate" consumption is generally defined as 25 grams of pure alcohol per day, equivalent to two or two and a half, 4-ounce glasses of wine per day.

The French locales with the highest wine consumption, such as Provence and other wine producing regions which consume less beer and spirits, had the lowest cirrhosis rates -- 7 to 14 per 100,000 -- putting them even lower than the U.S

The most recent study headed by Eric Rimm at the Harvard School of Public Health found cardiac protection at levels as high as 50 grams per day, although at the higher limits they also reported an increased risk of liver disease and of some cancers.

In fact, statistics pointing to these increases are often cited by alcohol control groups as reasons why people should not drink **any** alcohol. However, Dr. Ellison said that in essentially all studies, moderate drinkers have a significantly lower death rate (usually 20 to 40 percent less) **from all causes** than abstainers and even lower rates than heavy (5 to 6 drinks per day) drinkers. Dr. Ellison said that while the research is not conclusive, increased cancers and liver disease are associated with "especially heavy drinking and alcohol abuse but generally not increased with moderate wine consumption."

The reason for this is the relative rarity of liver disease compared with coronary artery disease. The World Health Organization's 1989 World Health Statistics Annual found in the United States that the death rate from cirrhosis of the liver was 17 per 100,000 while cardiovascular disease killed 464 per 100,000. By contrast, the same study shows France with almost double the cirrhosis rate -- 31 per 100,000 -- but with cardiovascular rates at only 310 per 100,000.

Using these figures, it is not hard to see that if the U.S. rates were normalized with those of France, 14 more people per 100,000 would die of cirrhosis, but 154 **fewer** people would die of cardiovascular disease, a net savings of 140 people per 100,000 population who would

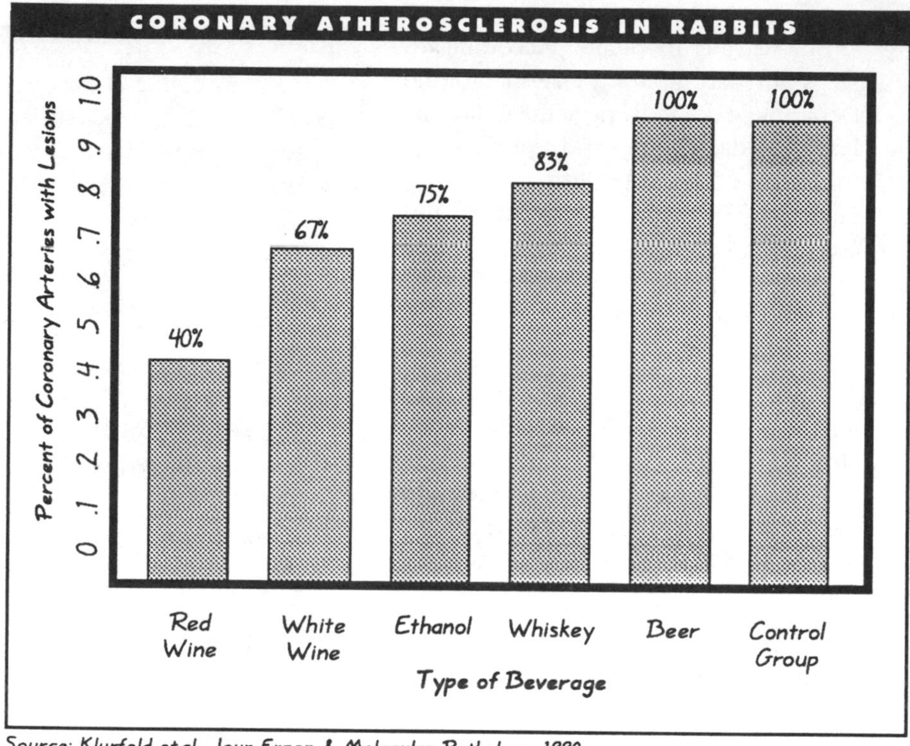

Source: Klurfeld et.al. Jour Exper. & Molecular Pathology. 1990

live longer in order to die later of something else (for, after all, the death rate is eventually 100 percent).

In fact the statistics also hide a striking pattern in the French cirrhosis rates. Dr. Renaud said that INSERM studied the rates on a regional basis and found the highest cirrhosis rates (50 to 100 per 100,000) in the northern regions of Alsace and Lorraine which have the highest consumption of beer and spirits.

However, the locales with the highest wine consumption, such as Provence and other wine producing regions which consume less beer and spirits, had the lowest cirrhosis rates -- 7 to 14 per 100,000 -- putting them even lower than the U.S.

Some people have questioned the wine versus other alcoholic beverages figures on socioeconomic grounds; research indicates that, at least in America, wine drinkers are better-educated, earn more money and are in a better position to eat healthier and get better medical care.

"There's no other drug that is so efficient (at preventing heart disease) as moderate intake of alcohol," said Dr. Renaud, who cautions against excessive consumption. "It has to be given at a proper dosage."

However, animal studies with rabbits have shown the same sort and degree of protective effects of alcohol as human studies. In a study published by researchers Klurfeld and Kritchevsky in the *Journal of Experimental and Molecular Pathology*, the following effects were observed (see next page):

As with cirrhosis, the increased risk of cancers, said Dr. Ellison, also seems connected more with abuse than with moderate use. In fact, red wine contains *quercetin*, a compound also found in garlic and onions which has been proven to exhibit strong **anti-cancer** effects. The research, however, is not yet advanced enough to draw any conclusions with regard to quercetin in wine.

There may be some connection between moderate alcohol consumption and an increase in breast cancer. According to Dr. Marton, a review of 24 major studies shows 12 finding no association between moderate consumption and breast cancer, and 12 which indicate there may be as much as a 4 percent increase in the lifetime risk of breast cancer. "Many of these studies," Dr. Marton said, "do not account for other factors (other than alcohol) that might affect the risk of cancer.

However, Dr. Marton said that even if you accept the worst-case studies as valid, a woman who drinks moderately must balance the 4 percent **increase** in the risk of getting breast cancer against the 10 to 20 percent **decrease** in risk of dying of heart disease - - a net positive effect of 6 to 14 percent.

"It's well documented that a moderate intake of alcohol prevents coronary heart disease by as much as 50 percent." —Dr. Serge Renaud, M.D.

"There's no other drug that is so efficient (at preventing heart disease) as moderate intake of alcohol," said Dr. Renaud, who cautions against excessive consumption. "It has to be given at a proper dosage."

Such proper dosages, according to Dr. Ellison, could produce this protective effect by increasing HDL lipoproteins (the "good" cholesterol) and decreasing LDL lipoproteins (the "bad" cholesterol). In addition, he said research also shows that alcohol decreases the tendency of blood to clot in arteries and increases fibrinolysis -- the ability to dissolve clots once they have formed.

In addition, he feels that three other factors may also contribute to alcohol's protective role. These possible (and he repeatedly emphasizes "possible") mechanisms may be that moderate alcohol consumption:

- ♥ Reduces the tendency of arteries to constrict during stress which decreases blood flow,
- ♥ Lowers blood pressure and
- ♥ Increases coronary artery diameter and blood flow.

But wine alone may not explain the French Paradox entirely. Dr. Ellison and others believe that the French diet may also play a substantial role.

The French eat more fresh fruits and vegetables which are fresher than American equivalents and more often consumed raw or with minimum cooking. This, Dr. Ellison and others feel, preserves vitamins that act as anti-oxidants which not only decrease the development of atherosclerosis (clogging/hardening of the arteries) but may also retard cancer development.

In addition, the French take more time with their meals which is not only a possible stress reducer, but may affect the absorption and metabolism of fats, insulin levels or the effects of fats on blood clotting.

Snacks also play a smaller dietary role in France. Dr. Ellison said that in a recent study he found that the French averaged 7.5 percent of their daily calories from snacks while Americans averaged 21 percent. This figure may be aggravated by high-fat American snacks and techno-foods.

> ***"Some French research shows that goose fat -- such as that found in foie gras -- may be less atherogenic since it contains more monounsaturated fats than other animal fats."***

The French diet also contains smaller portions of red meat which has much less fat than American meat.

Dairy food consumption also differs strikingly from the American patterns. The French consume their dairy products in the form of cheese, rather than whole milk. Dr. Renaud said his research indicates that the calcium in cheese may bind to the fat, making it less likely to be absorbed by the body. No such binding effect has been observed in whole milk, he said.

In addition to dairy fat, the French use more olive oil and goose fat than butter, lard or other animal fats. "This is most true in the south of France where heart disease is particularly uncommon," said Dr. Ellison. "Numerous studies have shown that olive oil is less atherogenic [less likely to cause hardening of the arteries]," he added. "Some French research shows that goose fat -- such as that found in foie gras -- **may** be less atherogenic since it contains more monounsaturated fats than other animal fats."

The role of dietary fat in the French Paradox has become somewhat controversial. One nutritionist, Marion Nestle, chair of the New York University Department of Nutrition, Food and Hotel Management, asserts that the data on lower French heart disease rates comes from a time period when the French were eating less fat than Americans and this accounts for much of their lower cardiovascular death rates; thus there is no paradox at all.

Nestle uses food supply data from the U.N.'s Food and Agriculture Organization (FAO) to support her claims. The supply numbers, she said, are produced by taking food production statistics, subtracting

Red wine contains** quercetin, **a compound also found in garlic and onions which has been proven to exhibit strong anti-cancer effects.

exports, adding imports and then dividing by the population to produce a per-capita consumption figure.

She said that these data indicate that the French diet has only caught up with the Americans' in the past decade. In 1961, she said, the French ate 28 percent of their calories from fat, increasing to 30 percent in 1965, to 34 percent in 1975, to 37 percent in 1985 and to 39 percent in 1988. By contrast, Americans first consumed 35 percent of their dietary calories from fat in 1923 and hit 42 percent in 1988.

Nestle admitted that the food production number is "not an absolutely accurate indicator of what people are actually eating" but that it provides a method which can be consistently applied over a period of many years. She said that variations in the methods of measuring actual consumption prevent this consistent approach.

Drs. Ellison and Renaud say they have based their research and calculations on (among many sources) actual consumption figures developed by the World Health Organization's (WHO) MONICA Project and feel that their numbers are sound.

This disagreement in historical data is important because several studies indicate that atherosclerosis may begin in early childhood. Thus, a 50-year-old's 1992 heart attack may have its roots in 1942. But researchers have not yet reconciled this data with numerous studies which indicate that switching to healthier, low-fat diets can affect the course of heart disease for people in their 40s and older. This means that even with a worst-case interpretation of the statistics, the French Paradox may be providing at least partial protection.

There is, however, no disagreement among the experts that the French traditional cuisine and wine consumption habits are eroding and becoming more like Americans. What's more, genetic factors cannot protect them from the ravages of techno-food, stress and unsound diets.

Drs. Ellison and Renaud (along with other researchers) say that while genetic factors are important in determining an individual's risk of heart disease, they apparently are not a factor in explaining the French Paradox. They cite numerous studies that show that people from the Mediterranean and other countries who immigrate to the U.S. soon lose the protective advantages of their native cuisine and lifestyles and begin suffering from the same dietary-related diseases that afflict Americans -- once they start to eat like Americans. Thus, as the French begin to eat more like Americans, they will begin to die like Americans -- increasingly of cardiovascular disease.

"If wine is ever found to contain a constituent protective against IHD (ischemic heart disease) then we consider it almost a sacrilege that this constituent be isolated. The medicine is already in a highly palatable form."

But, Dr. Ellison cautions, Americans shouldn't rush out and gorge themselves on wine and pate. Moderation, he cautions, is key. In addition, he said that American efforts to cut down on fats, eliminate smoking and engage in exercise should remain priorities. The key is not to adopt a new style of eating just for the sake of health, but because it tastes good and provides pleasure.

Dr. Ellison and others say that the pressures to be healthier -- to exercise, diet and eat right no matter what -- may produce unhealthy stresses of their own.

The tasty, enjoyable aspects of the healthy French way of eating are well illustrated by Peter Mayle, an English author and journalist who turned his back on his fat- and sugar-heavy native cuisine. In *Toujours Provence* (the sequel to *A Year In Provence*), Mayle writes of the seemingly limitless drinking of wine and pastis and says,

"It is impossible to live in France for any length of time and stay immune from the national enthusiasm for food, and who would want to? Why not make a daily pleasure out of a daily necessity? We have slipped into the gastronomic rhythm of Provence, taking advantage of the special offers provided by nature all through the year ... Meat everyday is a habit of the past. There is so much else: fish from the

Thus, as the French begin to eat more like Americans, they will begin to die like Americans -- increasingly of cardiovascular disease.

Mediterranean, fresh pasta, limitless recipes for those vegetables, breads, hundreds of cheeses.

"It may be the change in our diet and the way it is cooked, always in olive oil, but we have both lost weight."

Finally, a group of British scientists, who found protective effects from moderate wine consumption wrote in the respected British medical journal *Lancet*, "If wine is ever found to contain a constituent protective against IHD (ischemic heart disease) then we consider it almost a sacrilege that this constituent be isolated. The medicine is already in a highly palatable form."

TWO

Our Promise To You

We Want To Help You Prevent Heart Disease And Lead A Longer, More Disease-Free Life Without A Lifetime Of Deprivation And Bland Food

Your purchase of this book means that you're probably aware that heart disease kills more than 500,000 people in the United States every year. Death was the first symptom for 40 percent of those people. This insidious disease forever alters the lives of an additional one million heart attack survivors each year. Survivors and their families find their lives shaped by the brush with death even when recovery is "complete." Thousands whose recoveries are not so complete will face shortened life spans, with their remaining years plagued by pain, fear and disability.

Death is the first symptom for 40 percent of the people who die of heart disease.

"Oh!" These people say, "If only I could have prevented the disease in the first place!"

PROMISE #1: We will show you ways to dramatically decrease your chances of getting a heart attack.

Prevention is so important because, despite the dramatic decline in **deaths** from cardiovascular disease (about 40 percent in the U.S. in the past three decades), the **incidence** of heart attacks is roughly the same. Fewer people are dying mostly because medical treatment has improved, **not** because fewer people are getting sick.

What's more, the sophisticated medical treatments to save these people -- transplants, bypass surgery, angioplasty, clot-busting drugs -- are enormously expensive. They are frequently just temporary fixes, especially when the victims fail to make the eating, drinking and lifestyle changes that helped cause the disease in the first place.

Most people who fail to make these changes (either before or after a heart attack) do so because it requires radical alterations in their lifestyles involving extensive, time- consuming food preparation that, after all the effort, produces bland, unsatisfying meals.

Either consciously or subconsciously, many people fail to follow prevention techniques because they feel that a few more years of a life of deprivation may not be worth the effort.

PROMISE #2: We will show you how to eat healthy, delicious food that requires no special preparation, no hard-to- find foods and no deprivation.

In the United States people are working more hours and so turn to fast, frozen or prepared foods to salve the hunger in their stressed, time-pressed lives. The situation is aggravated because people think -- incorrectly we believe -- that they don't have time to prepare a tasty, healthy meal from fresh ingredients.

That's why every recipe or lifestyle change technique in this book will take less than 60 minutes to accomplish.

PROMISE #3: Everything we show you how to do in this book can be accomplished in less than 60 minutes out of your busy day.

This book was prompted by a gathering mountain of scientific research into a phenomenon known as "The French Paradox," which was dramatically reported on Nov. 17, 1991, on a segment of the CBS News program *60 Minutes*. Simply put, the French Paradox means that the French (and most other people in the Mediterranean region) have 40 percent fewer heart attacks than Americans although they:

- smoke tobacco prodigiously,
- exercise little,
- eat large amounts of fat,
- have the same, or slightly higher, blood cholesterol levels and
- spend far less per capita on health care.

Scores of research studies indicate that the French have fewer heart attacks because they:

- regularly drink moderate amounts of alcohol, particularly red wine, with meals,
- eat more fresh fruits and vegetables and
- take more time with their meals and with meal preparation.

PROMISE #4: We will show you how you can apply the French Paradox to your everyday life and increase your chances of living a longer, better, happier life.

We believe that the less you have to alter your life, the more likely you are to make the changes.

Old habits die hard, psychologists tell us, because the habits serve a purpose in your life. We realize that American society prevents most of us from living the lifestyle of a French or Italian or Greek peasant and their slower-paced lives filled with long midday meals and wine. But we will offer you solid, easily- accomplished ways of integrating important elements of this healthy lifestyle into your busy American life.

PROMISE #5: We will show you how to live, eat and drink healthier without disrupting your life

Our lives are uncertain in so many ways. We would love to know with certainty that if we do something or abstain from something that we will be healthier, live longer, avoid cancer, heart attacks and so forth.

But most scientific studies don't offer clear, black-and-white conclusions. They offer information based on the study of large numbers of individuals in a given population -- whether of mice or men and women. These studies are estimates based on effects of the studied population **as a whole** and cannot be applied with certainty to a given individual.

Whether these are studies to determine the effectiveness of a treatment, to determine the appropriate dose of a given antibiotic (or even common drugs like aspirin) or to determine which lifestyles are healthier, they are actually research- backed, highly educated guesses that the **chances are good** that a specific course of treatment will work.

People who regularly consume approximately two glasses of wine per day have as little as half the death rate from heart attacks *as either abstainers or heavy drinkers.*

Thus, your doctor cannot **guarantee** with 100 percent certainty that lowering your cholesterol will prevent a heart attack, that a particular antibiotic will cure your infection, that aspirin won't kill you, that angioplasty will cure your coronary artery blockage, or that you won't be the 1-in-10,000 who will die of a reaction to general anesthesia in a dentist's chair.

All a doctor or dentist -- or you -- can do is refer to the research and determine that, in the population studied, a given treatment has a stated chance of producing a desired result.

This means we know that large populations of people who take aspirin have an excellent chance of reducing pain; that studies of large numbers of people show that Tetracycline is effective in curing certain bacterial infection, and that population studies show that people who regularly consume approximately two glasses of wine per day have as little as half the death rate from heart attacks as either abstainers or heavy drinkers.

While engaging in these treatments or behaviors doesn't guarantee that your headache will be cured by aspirin or that moderate drinking will prevent your heart attack, the research does say that if you adopt them, you will place yourself in the same situation as the tested population and therefore increase your chances of benefiting.

In addition, studies are often flawed, incomplete or conflict with each other. In these cases, you must weigh the pluses and minuses of each to make an intelligent and informed decision.

PROMISE #6: We will help you interpret the studies and research so you can figure out for yourself what they really mean. We hope to better equip you to take charge of your own life and make your own health and lifestyle decisions.

There are many people in the government, in private anti-alcohol advocacy groups as well as some in the alcoholic beverage industry who have vested interests in twisting or hiding research data to support their own agendas. The general media's lack of time (or reluctance) to tell a complete story only makes things worse when you try to base your own lifestyle choices on flawed information.

We will give you some practical ways in which you can evaluate new medical research and determine who is trying to lie to you...and why.

To Think About

An exposition and critical review of the methods and assumptions used by the National Institute on Alcohol Abuse and Alcoholism (NIAAA) to estimate the economic costs of alcohol abuse have been interpreted as being flawed empirically and conceptually. *"This study concludes that these estimates are inaccurate and that they continually overstate actual costs."* Heien, D., and Pittman, D., "The Economic Costs of Alcohol Abuse: An Assessment of Current Methods and Estimates," Journal of Studies on Alcohol, September, p. 3, 1989.

Sidebar One

What Is Alcohol, Anyway?

Most people don't realize that their bodies contain scores of types of alcohols even if they've never taken a drink.

To an organic chemist, an alcohol is any compound with a *hydroxyl* group attached to a saturated carbon atom.

A "saturated" carbon atom is one which is attached to four other atoms; a hydroxyl group is the organic chemist's name for an "almost molecule" consisting of one oxygen and one hydrogen atom.

By this chemical definition, cholesterol is an alcohol; so are glycerol (a key part of triglycerides), Vitamin A, lactic acid (which builds up in your muscles following intense exercise), methanol (highly toxic, also known as methyl alcohol and wood alcohol), and sorbitol (which tastes sweet and may be marketed as a sugar substitute).

But what concerns us here is *ethyl* alcohol, also known as *ethanol.* It takes its name because a hydroxyl group is added to a saturated, two-carbon configuration which organic chemists call an ethyl group.

Ethanol is inescapable because all it takes to get fermentation started is sugar and yeast -- both of which are ubiquitous in our environment and food supply.

Take a molecule of glucose, add yeast and very quickly you get two molecules each of alcohol and carbon dioxide.

Primitive people never heard of Chardonnay or Miller Time, but they discovered that if they ate fruit, especially grapes, that was left too long in a warm spot, it would do funny things to their outlook on prehistoric life. All the yeasts necessary to ferment grapes actually grow on the skin of each grape. It's as if each grape wears a "Born To Ferment" tattoo.

The same fermentation will happen to apple juice, orange juice or other fruit juices and fruit left in your refrigerator. In fact, laboratory samplings of commonly consumed fruit juices and sugar- based soft drinks purchased from a supermarket (and tested right from the carton the day they were put

ALCOHOL IN FRUIT JUICES

Product	% alc. "Fresh"	% Alc. Day 3
Organic apple juice	<0.01	0.03
Minute Maid orange juice	0.11	0.18
Dole pineapple juice	0.08	0.34
Apple Time apple juice	0.10	0.34
Coca-Cola Classic	0.07	0.08
Minute Maid grape juice	0.06	W/A

Source: ETS LABS. 1992

on the store shelf) all showed measurable amounts of ethanol, up to 0.1 percent.

The amount of ethanol in some of the samples doubled or tripled after only three days in the refrigerator.

The fermentation used to produce wine, beer and spirits is much more carefully controlled and the particular species of yeast (called *strains*) are selected for their ability to produce desired tastes and other characteristics.

Fermentation and production methods vary greatly even among makers of each type of beverage, but each of the three main categories has its basic technique.

Wine is the easiest. The grapes are crushed and the juice drained into a container. Fermentation then begins with the natural yeasts or others added by the winemaker. Fermentation stops naturally when one of two things happens: (1) all the sugar is converted to alcohol, or (2) the alcohol content reaches a level (usually around 15 percent by volume) that kills the yeast.

The intense natural grape tastes and the minimum amount of manipulation required to make wine makes it the most intensely flavored of the three main categories of alcoholic beverages.

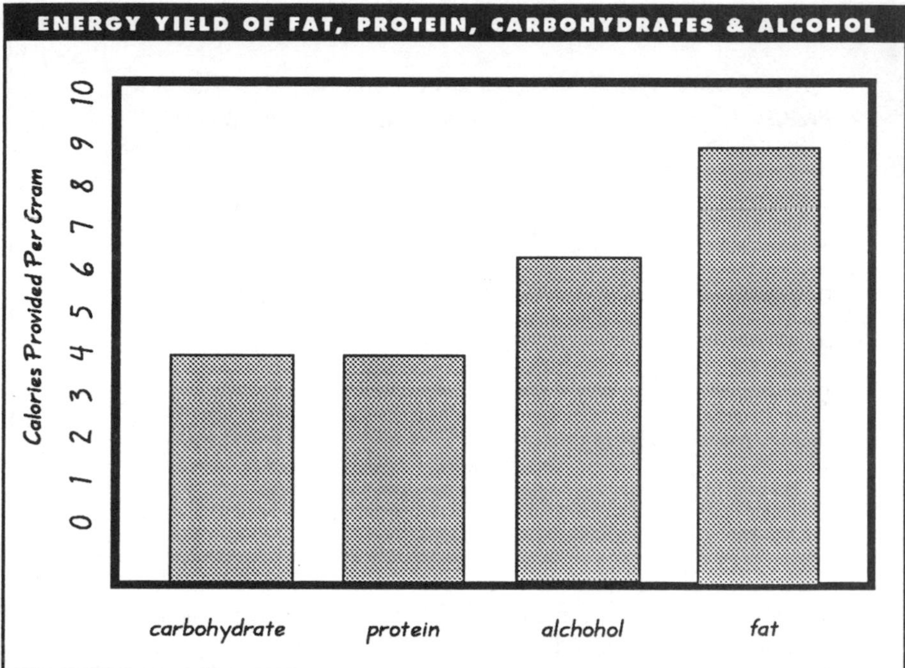

Fortified wines, dessert wines, ports and madeiras are usually made by adding grape brandy to partially fermented (and thus sweet) wines to increase alcohol content up to about 22 percent. However, some "late harvest" wines start out with very high sugar levels in the grapes and, with special strains of yeast, can be naturally fermented to produce both sweetness and higher alcohol.

Beer and distilled spirits made from grain and other starches are much more complicated. Starches are made up of long chains of sugars and must be "pre-digested" before yeast can ferment the sugars. Most grains used in beer and other liquor are allowed to germinate slightly to produce enzymes that liberate the sugars which are then converted to alcohol. American beer is usually about 3.5 percent alcohol; ales, stouts and malt liquors are usually higher -- normally up to about 8 to 10 percent.

The brewmaster helps impart

flavors to the beverage by adding hops and by various methods of toasting the grain. The resins leached from the hops also act as a preservative.

Distilled spirits are just that -- concentrated solutions of alcohol heated to a point where the alcohol boils off and is collected by a condenser. Some spirits are distilled more than once, thus increasing the alcohol content and further concentrating the faint flavors which survive the distillation process.

Spirits made with starches, which have little taste at all (like vodka) are infused with flavors by aging in wood or by adding other substances (like juniper berries in gin). The wood also helps take some of the rough edges off the high alcohol content which can run to 50 percent or more. Brandy and cognac are distilled from wine.

In general, the higher the alcohol content of a beverage, the more stable it is (that is, unlikely to spoil).

THREE

What's All The Fuss About?

The November 1991 segment of CBS's *60 Minutes* introduced millions of Americans to the cardio-protective effects of moderate alcohol consumption. But the phenomenon has been known since 1926 when a study of tuberculosis patients in a sanatorium found that patients who drank alcohol moderately had approximately half the death rate as those who abstained.

The U.S. government and the American medical establishment didn't rush to embrace this finding, conducted as it was, during the midst of Prohibition.

Medical science has progressed enormously since then with scores of university and hospital studies in the United States and abroad offering not just theories and hypotheses, but hard, reliable facts. Abstainers and heavy drinkers die sooner of all causes and are hit with crippling or lethal heart attacks at almost twice the rate as their moderately sipping neighbors.

Abstainers and heavy drinkers die sooner of all causes and are hit with crippling or lethal heart attacks at almost twice the rate as their moderately sipping neighbors.

Again, it's important to remember that alcohol **abuse** -- heavy, addictive consumption -- is a serious problem for society. An estimated 7 to 10 percent of Americans cannot consume alcohol moderately and should drink **none**. It's also important to remember that while moderate drinkers have a lower death rate from all causes, heavy drinkers are at increased risk for cancer, liver diseases, and accidents. Chronic heavy drinking also causes high blood pressure with a resulting increase in risk for heart disease.

"The epidemiological community has known for many years that moderate alcohol consumption is associated with lower cardiovascular mortality rates but has not publicized this fact, perhaps because of the fear that making a positive statement about drinking would lead to

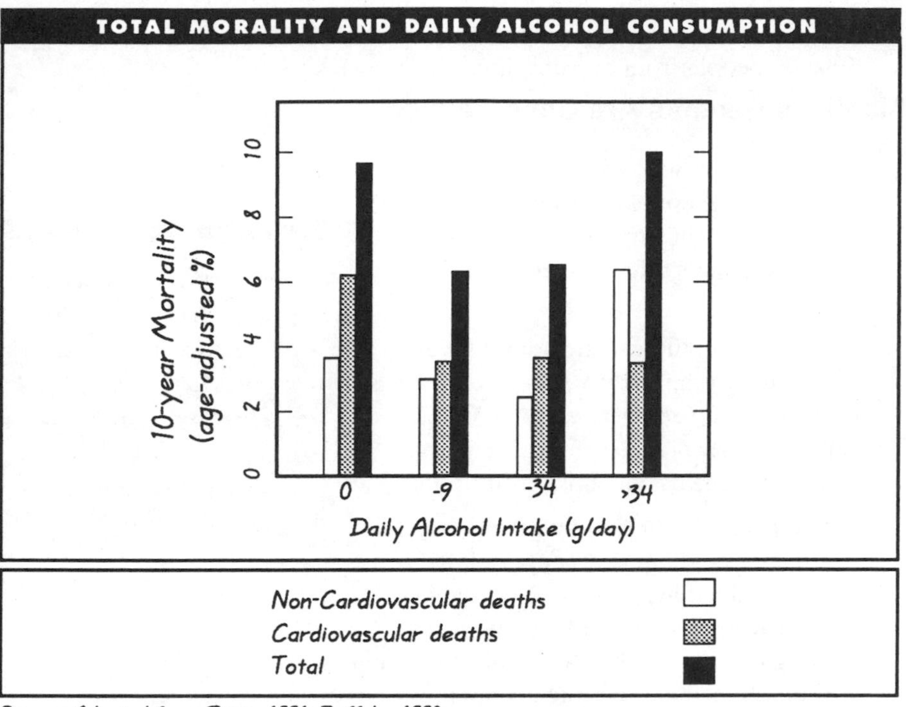

Source: Adapted from Rimm. 1991: Boffeha. 1990

greater abuse of alcohol," said Dr. Curtis Ellison, Chief of the Section of Preventive Medicine and Epidemiology at the Boston University School of Medicine in an editorial in the September 1990 issue of *Epidemiology.*

This fear, Dr. Ellison said, is not supported by scientific or medical fact. "People who abuse alcohol are addictive personalities and they will abuse regardless of the medical advice given," he said.

Researchers point to alcoholics who will drink perfume, mouthwash and other sources of alcohol when beverage alcohol is unavailable.

But for the other 90 to 93 percent of Americans, proper knowledge and application of the scientific facts might **save more than 200,000**

people every year from dying of heart attacks and save another 500,000 people from even having a heart attack.

Alcohol's Benefits Are Dose Related

We now know as much or more about the cardio-protective effects of moderate alcohol consumption as we do about aspirin's role in reducing heart attacks or fiber's role in decreasing colon cancer.

The J-shaped curve means that the effects -- good or bad -- are *dose-related*: ***the right amount is good for you while too little or too much can be unhealthy.***

Numerous studies, including several conducted in the early 1990s, reveal the existence of a *J-shaped curve* (sometimes called a *U-shaped curve*) which graphs death rates against alcohol consumption.

The J-shaped curve shows that overall death rates begin to drop in people who drink moderately. The curve reaches bottom at some point and then begins to rise again as alcohol consumption increases. With increasing consumption, the death rate eventually draws even with abstainers and then continues upward, with heavy drinkers having the highest death rates of all.

This J-shaped curve is a fairly common one in medicine and is associated with a wide variety of substances which become harmful if too little or too much of it is consumed. Vitamin A, for instance, causes disease when it becomes scarce; yet it is toxic when too much is consumed. Most life-saving pharmacueticals exhibit this same J-shaped behavior: too little is unhealthy, too much is dangerous. This is true whether the pharmacueticals are antibiotics, cholesterol-lowering drugs, hypertension medicine, ulcer medication and so on.

The J-shaped curve means that the effects -- good or bad -- are *dose-related*: the right amount is good for you while too little or too much can be unhealthy.

While alcohol is not a pharmacuetical to be prescribed as medicine, you need to recognize that its effects are dose related. To obtain the healthiest results, your consumption needs to be moderate. As you will learn, the definition of "moderate" drinking varies from study to study, ranging from one to five "drinks" per day (a drink being equivalent to 10 to 12 grams of pure alcohol -- roughly a four- to five-ounce glass of table wine, one beer or one mixed drink). Most medical experts say that one to three drinks per day is the most responsible and acceptable definition of "moderate."

Where's The Evidence Of Cardio-Protective Effects?

More than two dozen hospital and university studies confirm the cardio-protective effects of moderate alcohol consumption in both men and women. One of the most recent was conducted by a research team headed by Eric Rimm at the Harvard University School of Public Health. The study, published in August 1991 in the respected British medical journal, *Lancet*, found that male physicians who drank, on average, one-half to one drink per day had 21 percent less coronary artery disease (CAD) than abstainers. Put another way, their *relative risk (RR)* was 0.79 compared to abstainers at 1.00.

The relative risk continued to drop with increased consumption. Men who consumed one to one and a half drinks per day reduced their CAD risk by 32 percent (RR=0.68; one and a half to three drinks per day reduced the risk by 27 percent (RR=0.73); three to four and a half per day reduced it by 43 percent (RR=0.57) and those drinking more than four and a half drinks per day reduced CAD risk by 59 percent (RR=0.41).

While the heart attack risk at the higher levels may seem attractive to some, this level is the beginning of heavy drinking (and perhaps abuse) and carries with it an increasing risk of other diseases.

Another landmark study of the health benefits of moderate alcohol consumption was published in the September 1990 issue of *Epidemiology* by Paolo Boffetta of the American Cancer Society and Lawrence Garfinkel of the International Agency for Research on Cancer, Lyon, France. Their study confirmed the J- shaped curve, but found somewhat lower protective effects from moderate consumption (perhaps due to under-reporting of consumption by participants or because they used a different way of categorizing consumption).

Using abstainers as a reference (RR = 1.00) they found that the RR for heart disease was 0.86 for occasional drinkers, 0.79 for those drinking one drink per day, 0.80 for those drinking two drinks per day and 0.83 for those drinking three drinks per day. The cardio-protective effects continued with increased drinking but began to decrease again for people drinking five or more drinks per day.

The relative risk (RR) of all causes of death was 0.88 for occasional drinkers, 0.84 for those drinking one drink per day, 0.93 for those drinking two drinks per day and 1.02 for those drinking three drinks per day.

An intelligent decision on whether something is fact or hypothesis can only be made by considering the* overall body of evidence *-- which is just another way of saying that a single study does not make for scientific fact.

One reason why the protective effects were smaller in their study than in other research can be found in Boffetta and Garfinkel's discussion of their research subjects. They emphasized that their study was of middle-aged men (40 to 59 years old) aging over time. "Therefore it can be expected that alcohol intake was also reduced during the follow-up period; if this is true...the present estimates will represent an underestimation of the true effects of alcohol drinking on coronary heart disease mortality,"

The Boffetta and Garfinkel study also found slight **decreases** in total cancers and accidents as well as the expected **increases** in suicide and liver cirrhosis. It's significant that some studies do not find an increase in suicides while others do.

Unfortunately, it's the nature of scientific research to find conflicting data. This is because small (or unaccounted for) variations in the methods of doing the research or analyzing the data can bias the outcome. Because of this, an intelligent decision on whether something is fact or hypothesis can only be made by considering the **overall body of evidence** -- which is just another way of saying that a single study does not make for scientific fact.

This book will present as **fact** only those conclusions based on **multiple confirming studies** conducted by respected organizations and a variety of different researchers. To do otherwise -- to try and base a conclusion on a single study -- is naive, scientifically unsound and intellectually dishonest. The studies presented in this book to illustrate **fact** (such as the ones you've read so far in this chapter) will be those representative of the overall body of evidence.

Flawed Studies?

Some of the older studies have been attacked by critics who charged that the results were biased because the abstainers studied included many people who were not drinking because they were already in bad health, or were possibly abstaining alcoholics.

> ***"the inverse relation between alcohol consumption and risk of coronary artery disease is causal."***

The Rimm study at Harvard was one of the first (but not the only one) to study this possibility and to correct for it in the analysis. The study concluded that excluding abstainers with pre-existing conditions did not alter the J-shaped curve or the conclusion that "the inverse relation between alcohol consumption and risk of coronary artery disease is causal."

Other critics of the J-shaped curve have suggested that people who drink alcohol are all somehow different or all engage in some other activity that accounts for the cardio-protective effect.

Numerous studies have eliminated education, race, cigarette smoking habits, coffee drinking and others as possible factors. Several of the important studies in this regard have been done by Dr. Arthur L. Klatsky, M.D., at the Kaiser Permanente Medical Center in Oakland, Calif. One of his major articles, published in the *American Journal of Cardiology* in 1986, corrects for these factors and "supports the view that alcohol protects against CAD."

Additional proof regarding other socio-economic factors, such as access to medical care, diet, income and personal habits, comes from

RISK FACTORS FOR HEART DISEASE

Behavior	Average factor of increase (Over person without behavior, factor will vary with degree of behavior)
High blood pressure	2.1X (times higher)
High cholesterol	2.4X
Smoking	2.5X
Sedentary lifestyle	1.9X
Alcohol abstinence or abuse	1.5X
Being male (compared with pre-menopausal women)	3.0X

Source: Adapted from "Physical Activity and the Incidence of Coronary Artery Disease" from the U.S Centers for Disease Control.

laboratory experiments conducted with rabbits at The Wistar Institute in Philadelphia. They found that in a genetically matched group of animals, those fed alcohol had up to 60 percent less coronary artery disease than rabbits who had no alcohol.

So Where's The Paradox?

As you read in Chapter One, the French (and most people around the Mediterranean) flout the laws of accepted medical knowledge with heavy cigarette smoking, high fat consumption and a relative lack of exercise.

Yet they live longer and suffer only one half as many heart attacks as Americans, despite the fact that their cholesterol levels are approximately equal to ours. **That's** the paradox that flies in the face of conventional medical wisdom.

Conventional medical wisdom's reluctance to cope with the beneficial effects of moderate alcohol consumption is also the reason that it took so long for scientific and medical research institutions to accept alcohol's role in keeping people heart healthy despite other bad habits.

Of all the factors considered, increased alcohol consumption had a stronger link to decreasing heart attack deaths than did decreased fat consumption or cigarette smoking.

Another key study linking moderate alcohol consumption, particularly wine, with cardio-protective effects, was published in 1979 in the *Lancet* and has been subsequently corroborated by data gathered over the past 12 years. That study, led by A.S. St. Leger of the British Medical Research Council's Epidemiology Unit in Cardiff, studied ischemic heart disease (IHD) deaths in 18 developed countries to determine what factors were associated with the deaths.

As expected, they found significantly strong positive associations between smoking and deaths from all causes. (A positive association means that as the behavior or other measured factor increases, the death rate rises; a negative association means that the death rate decreases as the measured behavior increases.)

They also found strong positive associations between IHD deaths and total fat intake and also total calorie intake.

Surprisingly, they found **no** strong association between IHD deaths and such health-service factors as the number of doctors and nurses per 100,000 population.

The St. Leger team also found a number of strongly negative associations with IHD deaths. The IHD death rates were lower as the per capita gross national product and population density increased. But the most surpring finding was that the strongest negative association in the entire study was the link with alcohol consumption. In other words, of all the factors considered, increased alcohol consumption had a stronger link to decreasing heart attack deaths than did decreased fat consumption or cigarette smoking.

This is not to say that smoking or high fat consumption is safe if you drink alcohol because people who engage in those risky behaviors have a significantly higher risk of dying sooner and having more heart attacks than moderate drinkers who eat smart and don't smoke.

The St. Leger study is one of the few to distinguish among consumption of wine, beer and distilled spirits. While their study strongly linked total alcohol consumption with decreased IHD deaths, according to the published study, "This is shown to be wholly attributable to wine consumption."

This observation has been somewhat inconsistent in the total body of research where some studies have given the edge to beer or spirits and others to wine. If wine is found to have an edge in this regard, scientists say it may not be due to an intrinsic difference among the beverage types, but be due more to the fact that wine is more often consumed with meals than the other two types of beverage.

To Think About:

"Wine is one of the oldest beverages known to man [or woman]. Written records dating back 4,000 years refer to the dietary and therapeutic uses of wine. It has been attractive to man as food, as a medicine, as a part of various religious and ritual ceremonies throughout the world, and as an important element in social life. In light of its ancient history, it is not surprising that many of the healthful effects of wine have become legendary." — McDonald, J. and Sheldon M., M.D., "Wine Versus Ethanol in Human Nutrition." The American Journal of Clinical Nutrition, No. 29, October, 1976, p. 1093.

Sidebar Two

What's a Drink Anyway?

This is a question very much like "what's blue?" It depends very much on who's asking the question and how good the memory is of the person who answers it.

Most scientific studies on the health effects of alcohol have generally defined a "drink" as 8 to 12 grams of alcohol.

What does this mean to your consumption patterns?

- ♥ A four-ounce glass of table wine (12 percent alcohol) has about 14 grams of alcohol.
- ♥ A 12-ounce serving of American beer (3.2 percent alcohol) has about 11.5 grams of alcohol.
- ♥ A mixed drink with a jigger (1.5 ounces) of 80-proof spirits has about 18 grams of alcohol.

As you'll read in other chapters of this book, there are significant differences among the health effects associated with these three basic types of beverage alcohol. Drinking patterns and the composition of the beverage itself both play a role.

But human behavior frequently confounds the precision of science, especially when it comes to alcohol which, in American society, is emotionally laden and (for some people) connected with guilt and sin. Epidemiological studies rely on people to remember things like drinking patterns and report them to researchers.

Scientists say that the emotional baggage of alcohol, combined with memory flaws and selective recall, results in **under**- reporting of alcohol consumption. People tend to report drinking less frequently than they actually do and they report drinking smaller amounts than they actually consume. This means that a "drink" is probably somewhat larger than the scientific definition. However, if you stick to the scientific definition, then you probably have a safety margin built in.

FOUR

What's Wrong With Intervention? Plenty!

The intervention-oriented medical system in the United States leads physicians to think more in terms of treatment than prevention. But don't blame everything on the physician. After all, they're just following the lead of a society and its government that is addicted to the quick fix rather than long- term prevention. We want to **control** high cholesterol with drugs rather than prevent it; fix faulty hearts with clot busting drugs, bypass surgery, angioplasty, fiber-optic laser clot zappers and the like; develop "magic bullet" drugs to cure cancer.

Much of the risk (if not almost all) of coronary artery disease can be reduced with a proper diet, exercise, decreasing stress and moderate consumption of alcohol.

Despite this, most cancers and heart disease result from diet and lifestyle factors that can be altered to **prevent** disease. Much of the risk (if not almost all) of coronary artery disease can be reduced with a proper diet, exercise, decreasing stress and moderate consumption of alcohol.

Likewise, controlling cancer is mostly in your hands. The *Journal of the National Cancer Institute* estimates that 35 percent of cancers can be attributed to diet and 30 percent to tobacco -- that means that **you can prevent about two-thirds of all cancers.**

The Pitfalls of Intervention

Despite the billions of dollars spent on intervention, it remains an appallingly rotten alternative to prevention. Intervention:

- comes too late for many people,
- frequently doesn't work,
- is frequently not permanent, and
- often has serious side effects.

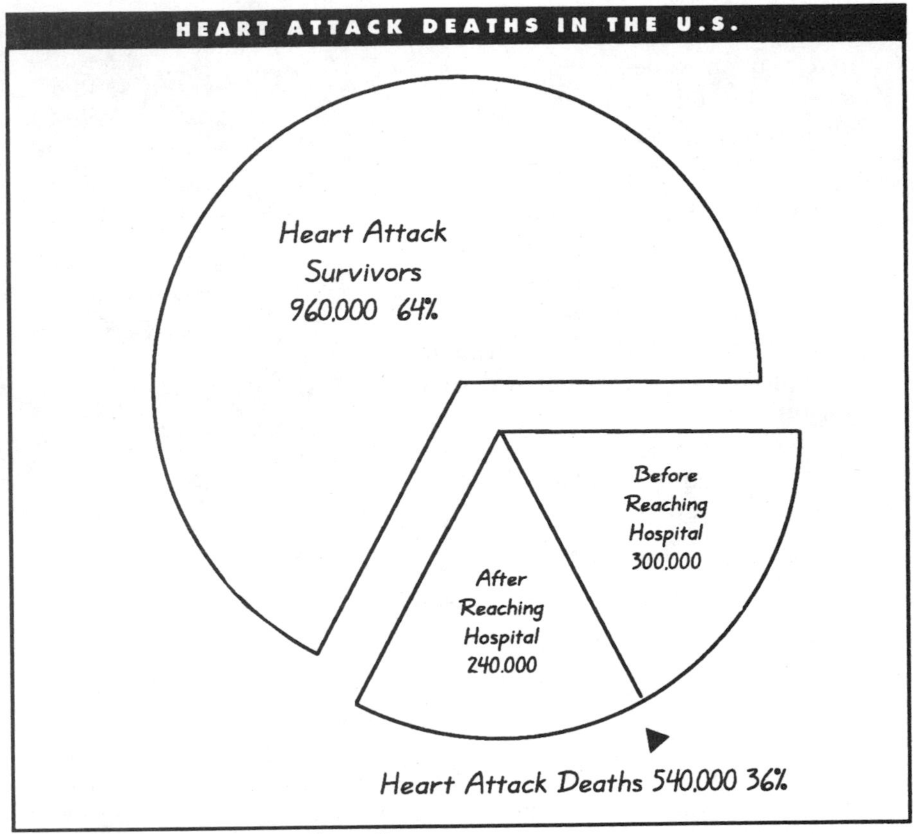

Source: U.S. Dept of Health and Human Services

Intervention comes too late for 18 percent of people whose first symptom of heart disease is death.

Intervention frequently doesn't work. About 350,000 coronary artery bypass graft surgeries are performed in the U.S. each year and a like number of balloon angioplasties.

Bypass surgery involves taking an artery from one part of the body, usually the leg, and grafting it to the blocked artery to bypass the blockages. Angioplasty involves placing a tiny balloon at the site of the artery blockage and inflating it to increase the diameter.

The lack of success for cancer intervention varies with the type of cancer, but the death rate for smokers with lung cancer, even with treatment, is almost 100 percent.

Intervention frequently is not permanent. About 50 percent of bypassed arteries clog up again after five years and 80 percent after seven years. One third of arteries treated with balloon angioplasty clog up within **four to six months**. The death rate from a second or third round of bypass surgery or angioplasty can be double or triple the first risk.

About 50 percent of bypassed arteries clog up again after five years and 80 percent after seven years...The death rate from a second or third round of bypass surgery or angioplasty can be double or triple the first risk.

Five-year survival rates for cancer can be depressingly low, despite the pain and horrors of surgery, radiation and chemotherapy.

Intervention often has side effects. The drugs used to lower blood pressure have a wide range of side effects including impotence in men, depression, fatigue, and blood cell malfunctions. The commonly used cholesterol-lowering drugs can cause liver damage, gastrointestinal tract disorders, cataracts, nausea and other problems. Many drugs used to help prevent clots dramatically increase the risk of hemorrhagic strokes. The radiation and chemotherapy drugs used to treat many cancers can cause severe nausea and may themselves, years later, cause other types of cancer.

Intervention is enormously expensive. An uncomplicated coronary artery bypass operation can cost $30,000, an angioplasty, $7,500. Estimates from the government and from insurance companies vary, but in 1990, approximately $78 billion was spent treating heart disease and at least $8 billion of that was spent on bypass surgery alone.

Drug therapy also comes dearly: the most common cholesterol-lowering drug, *Lovastatin*, costs $2,000 to $3,000 per year for one person.

This represents an incredible drag on our economy and the health care system. A universal health care system for **all** Americans could be

A universal health care system for all Americans could be funded with the interevention treatment money spent on preventable heart disease and cancers.

funded with the interevention treatment money spent on preventable heart disease and cancers.

The U.S. health care system is stacked against prevention. In his book, *Reversing Heart Disease*, Dr. Dean Ornish, M.D., states the problem eloquently, "The third-party reimbursement system (health insurance, Medicare etc.) encourages the use of drugs and surgery rather than health education ... If I perform a balloon angioplasty on a patient, the insurance company will pay at least $7,500. If I spend the same amount of time teaching a heart patient about nutrition and stress management techniques, the insurance company will pay no more than $150. If I spend that time teaching a well person how to *stay* healthy, the insurance company will not pay at all."

To Think About

'The compound known as quercetin is one of nature's most potent anticancer agents. It is found in such foods as onions, broccoli, squash and red grapes... when the quercetin-sugar bond is broken, such as in fermentation of grape juice to wine, quercetin is liberated... Much the same process occurs in the human gut and the similarity may be what makes quercetin one of nature's most potent anticarcinogens." Leighton, T. , U.C. Berkeley Professor of Microbiology

FIVE

Aging Gracefully Through The Years

A person who reaches age 65 today can expect to live at least another 17 years. But that quantity of life may be at the expense of its quality. Many older people question the wisdom of life extended by invasive technology; robbed of independence and dependent on others for basic functions like bathing, eating, using the toilet or transferring from a bed to a chair and back.

Because of this, more and more people are asking how they can increase their chances of enjoying the additional years by staying healthy and aging gracefully.

> ***People who drank alcohol moderately (1 to 60 drinks per month) were 3.1 times more likely to age successfully than abstainers.***

A landmark study examined the factors that could predict healthy aging; almost 7,000 people in Alameda County, Calif. participated over a 20 year period from 1965-1984. The study, conducted by Dr. Jack M. Guralnik, M.D., of the U.S. National Institute on Aging and George A. Kaplan of the California Department of Health Services, was published in the *American Journal of Public Health* in June 1989.

The paper focused on people who were 65 to 89 years old in 1984. The study found that, of the original group, 41 percent had died before 1984 and 12.7 percent were in a "high-function" group. "High-function" was defined as being able to handle the basics of daily living plus such physical activities as:

- climbing stairs or walking one-half mile
- gardening
- shopping
- walking, swimming or other sports exercise and
- vigorous exercise (jogging, bicycling, tennis, dancing).

The factors which predict successful aging offer both optimism (because of those which can be influenced by an individual) and pessimism (because of societal and financial pressures not so easily addressed by individuals).

FACTORS AFFECTING SUCCESSFUL AGING

		high function vs. deceased odds ration (95% CI)	High function vs. Low/moderate function odds ration (95% CI)
Demographic Model			
Age (10 years)	Younger/Older	5.1 (3.2, 8.0)	1.5 (1.0, 2.3)
Sex	Male/Female	5.0 (0.3, 0.8	1.2** (0.7, 1.9)
Race	Not-black/Black	4.1 (1.4, 12.4)	3.1 (1.1, 9.3)
Family Income	Very adequate-adequate/ Marginal/inadequate	4.9 (3.0, 8.2)	3.1 (1.4, 10.2)
Chronic Conditions Model			
High Blood Pressure	No/Yes	6.7 (1.9, 23.8)	4.1** (1.2, 14.1)
Arthritis	No/Yes	2.4 (1.1, 5.3)	3.0 (1.4, 6.5)
Back Pain	No/Yes	1.9 (1.0, 3.7)	2.0 (1.1, 3.6)
Health Practices Model			
Smoking	Past-Never /Current	6.1 (3.3, 8.3)	2.2** (1.3, 3.8)
Relative Weight	Moderate/Other	2.6 (1.1, 6.1)	2.4 (1.1, 5.1)
Alcohol Consumption	1-60/None	3.1 (1.5, 6.5)	2.2 (1.1, 4.4)
	1-60/>60	2.5 (0.7, 8.2)	1.3 (0.4, 4.0)

*Odds ratios adjusted for age, race, sex, baseline functional status and all variables in model.

**For this variable, the ratio for high function vs low/moderate function is signicantly from the odds ratio for high function.

Source: Guralnik. Amer. Jour. Public health. 1989

High-function people -- the 12.7 percent who had aged successfully when examined in 1984 -- were the ones who (in 1965):

- had adequate incomes,
- were not African Americans,
- had normal blood pressure,
- had no arthritis,
- had no back pain,
- did not smoke,
- had moderate weight and
- were **moderate** consumers of alcohol.

It's an indictment of the inequities of American society that people who were not African Americans were 4.1 times more likely to be successful agers. Likewise, those with adequate incomes were 4.9 times more likely to age successfully.

People with normal blood pressure were 6.7 times more likely to be very active; those with no arthritis, 2.4 times and those with no back pain, 1.9 times more likely.

It's no surprise that cigarette smokers were 6.1 times more likely to be dead or fail to make the high-function group.

People with moderate weight (defined as less than 10 percent under or 30 percent over the Metropolitan Life Insurance height/weight table) were 2.6 times more apt to age successfully.

Those who drank alcohol moderately (1 to 60 drinks per month) were 3.1 times more likely to age successfully than abstainers. Moderate drinkers were also 2.5 times as likely to age successfully as heavy drinkers.

Sidebar Three

Beware of "Popular" Alcohol Advice

Occasionally, you'll read quotes in this book that came from other general interest health books. On the whole, those books are accurate and very helpful. But when it comes to alcohol, they sometimes let inaccurate, outdated or out-of-context information slip into their texts.

Because you may buy those books and find their alcohol information at odds with this one, the following section examines their quotes and then provides you with the correct information. While these are exact quotes from books in print, the specific title is not mentioned because there's no reason to cast doubt on the other fine information they impart.

THE QUOTE: *"More careful analyses of the studies cited above* [showing moderate drinkers to have lower death rates than abstainers or heavy drinkers] *reveal that many of the people who didn't drink at all chose not to drink because a number of them were in ill health or were recovering alcoholics."*

THE FACTS: This criticism was first raised in 1988 and all of the studies conducted since then, including the 15 published in 1990 and 1991, correct for this possibility. It does not at all alter the findings that moderate consumers of alcohol live longer than abstainers or heavy drinkers.

THE QUOTE: *"One reason why people who drink 'moderately' may live longer is that they have more social support than others who do not drink ... I suspect that the same benefits would result from having social support in activities not centered around alcohol."*

THE FACTS: What this author "suspects" is not only unproven in humans, it is directly disproven by animal studies. As cited in another chapter in this book, rabbits fed water, ethanol diluted with water, beer, spirits, red and white wine revealed that the rabbits getting only water had far more atherosclerotic lesions in their coronary arteries than the other rabbits. Those rabbits who fared best were the ones fed red wine, followed by those fed white wine. The animal studies pretty well eliminate socio-economic factors.

THE QUOTE: *"Alcohol has a direct, toxic effect on the heart."*

THE FACTS: This is true only for blood alcohol concentration levels reached by sustained heavy drinking and abuse.

THE QUOTE: *"Drinking less than one drink per day has been found to double the risk of hemorrhagic stroke."*

THE FACTS: While this has been found in some -- but not all -- studies, hemorrhagic strokes are rare compared with heart disease. Moreover, alcohol consumption may help prevent occlusive strokes, which occur nine to ten times as often as hemorrhagic strokes. The fact that strokes are relatively rare compared with coronary artery disease counts for the overall lower death rates **from all causes** for moderate drinkers.

THE QUOTE: *"Alcohol is a major factor in most accidents at work and at home."*

THE FACTS: Simply incorrect. There are no data to support this. In fact, data **do** say that most accidents are caused by human carelessness, not alcohol. Moderate drinkers miss fewer days of work than abstainers.

THE QUOTE: *"Somewhere between 50 and 80 percent of all fatal traffic accidents are alcohol-related."*

THE FACTS: Each death from drunk driving is doubly tragic because it is entirely preventable. **Do not drink and drive.** The U.S. National Highway Traffic Safety Administration (NHTSA) says that approximately 45 to 50 percent of all traffic fatalities are alcohol-related. Alcohol-related means that alcohol was found in **anyone** in the car. NHSTA figures indicate that alcohol may **cause** about half of all alcohol-related accidents; in other words, alcohol causes about a quarter of all traffic fatalities. While significantly lower than the popular wisdom, this figure is unacceptably high because it is entirely preventable.

Of people arrested for drunken driving, only 2 percent reported drinking wine; 54 percent drank beer; 23 percent liquor and the remainder a mixture of drinks, according to the U.S. Department of Justice, Bureau of Justice Statistics' 1988 publication, *Special Report: Drunk Driving* .

THE QUOTE: *"There are two types of HDL [good cholesterol]: HDL2 and HDL3. HDL2 helps to protect against coronary heart disease, but HDL3 does not. Alcohol raises HDL3."*

THE FACTS: While alcohol does raise HDL3 more than HDL2, both types of HDL protect against coronary artery disease.

THE QUOTE: *"That alcoholic nightcap might actually result in sleep problems."*

THE FACTS: While heavy drinking can result in sleep disturbances, moderate consumption does not.

THE QUOTE: *"Alcohol raises blood pressure in those trying to control their hypertension."*

THE FACTS: Moderate consumption can actually lower blood pressure; heavy drinkers tend to have hypertension.

THE QUOTE: *"It appears that any alcohol consumption, but especially three, four or more drinks daily, leads to enlargement of the heart."*

THE FACTS: One study (the Framingham study) has indicated that steady use of alcohol has a dose-related effect on heart size. While moderate consumption can decrease blood pressure and help protect the coronary arteries from atherosclerosis, heavy drinking (more than five drinks per day) can have unhealthy consequences. But even heavy drinking has a relatively small effect on the heart -- less than the effect of smoking, high blood pressure or exercise, all of which enlarge the heart. Chronic alcoholics can develop pathological heart enlargement over many years.

To Think About

"Over half (52%) of the hospitals in the top 65 metropolitan areas of the U.S. offer a wine service to their patients." A Survey of Wine Service in Hospitals in the Top Metropolitan Areas of the United States, Matheson and Matheson, Inc., San Francisco, p. 1, 1985.

SIX

Is It The Wine Or The Food? Yes...And No

While kicking tobacco addiction still remains the single most effective way to avoid heart disease, medical and scientific research point directly to:

- moderate, regular wine consumption with meals,
- moderate exercise and
- the consumption of low-fat, healthy foods -- especially fruits and vegetables,

as the most identifiable pro-active factors in reducing the chances of having a heart attack. Diet is also crucial in reducing the risks of getting other serious diseases like cancer.

But forgotten by Americans, who like quick, easy fixes to problems, is the pattern of consumption. And **the pattern of eating and drinking may be as important for health as what is eaten or drunk**.

> **Moderation** ***is frequently ignored by Americans who feel that if a little of something is good for you, then a*** **lot** ***must be better.***

In addition to consumption patterns, **moderation** is frequently ignored by Americans who feel that if a little of something is good for you, then a **lot** must be better. We all know people who believe that if slim (or bulked up) is healthy, then really slim/bulked up is even better. Regardless of the behavior, Americans seem driven to excess.

Psychiatrists and other researchers are increasingly learning that the near-obsessive attitudes that drive these behaviors create an unhealthy stress that may negate whatever benefits might otherwise have been achieved.

Here are some of the moderation and pattern-related facts and hypotheses that scientists feel help explain the French Paradox. It's important to remember that **a scientific hypothesis is not yet proven** but is the formulation of a conclusion based on (and not conflicting with) existing research. These hypotheses are first attempts to explain the scientific mechanisms behind some observed **facts**.

FACT #1: The French and Mediterranean people eat more vegetables and fruits than Americans; they eat them fresher and more often eat them raw or with less cooking.

BACKGROUND FACTS: This practice preserves vitamins (most notably Vitamins C and E and beta-carotene which are anti- oxidants) and which are thought to decrease the development of atherosclerosis and some cancers.

DISCUSSION: Adequate consumption of fresh fruits and vegetables is important, not only for the vitamins and minerals they contain, but also for the fiber they add to the diet. In addition, nutritionists and diet researchers increasingly believe that the "active ingredient" in a particular food (such as sulforaphane in broccoli, a potential cancer inhibitor) may not perform as promised when isolated from other component organic chemicals in the food.

Eating fresh fruits and vegetables (or fresh frozen which are very close in nutritional content) not only tastes better and is more fun than taking a supplement, it can be healthier.

LIFESTYLE TIP

Cook vegetables in your microwave oven. Put them in glass loaf or baking dishes and cover with a thick, microwave- suitable plastic wrap to keep in steam. Wrap large vegetables, like corn, individually in plastic wrap.

But taking fresh foods and cooking the life out of them defeats the purpose. It's been known for decades that the over-cooked styles of American food destroy many of the healthy nutrients and leave many more leached out in the cooking water.

The French and Mediterranean styles of cooking leave vegetables bright in color, firm and full of nutrients.

Fortunately, vegetables are tailor-made for microwave preparation which cooks vegetables quickly throughout, usually without added water.

FACT #2: French and Mediterranean meals last longer than American meals.

HYPOTHESIS: Longer meals slow the absorption and metabolism of fats, which may affect insulin levels and the effects of fats on blood platelets.

HYPOTHESIS: Longer meals decrease emotional stress by providing a break from daily events and by fostering conversation and human interaction.

LIFESTYLE TIP

When you buy frozen vegetables, avoid the processed techno-food varieties which usually contain added fats, preservatives, salt and other undesirable ingredients.

DISCUSSION: The human body has a remarkable ability to cope with tens of thousands of chemical compounds ranging from the healthy to the toxic. Small amounts of toxins, for example, can be scavenged, neutralized and excreted by the liver. But if the blood concentration of these chemicals increases too fast or reaches too high a concentration, the liver -- or other mechanisms -- become overwhelmed and health suffers.

Fat is needed in the human diet, but at far smaller concentrations than are normally found in the American diet -- or the French and Mediterranean diet for that matter. Like fat, many other healthful compounds -- ranging from Vitamin A and aspirin to alcohol and most therapeutic drugs -- can be toxic when the doses rise too high.

The fast, on-the-run meals consumed by Americans are usually very high in fat and sugar, causing insulin levels to skyrocket. Scientists have found that bouncing insulin levels (like those found in diabetics who take their insulin via syringe rather than by implanted pump) damage many of the body's tissues, especially blood vessels, and alter the way that cells metabolize food.

Insulin damage may promote the build-up of cholesterol in the artery walls leading to atherosclerosis.

LIFESTYLE TIP

Set aside at least one evening every week for family dinner; sit around the table and talk -- no television. Make this dinner an inviolable ritual by scheduling it for the same time and day of the week. More evenings are better, but one is a start. Make a rule that no activities are scheduled for after dinner to relieve the temptation to eat and run. Your children learn from you; what you teach them about lifestyle now can save them from a heart attack when they're your age.

In addition, high concentrations of fats in the blood may also increase the stickiness of platelets which promotes clotting.

Finally, some scientists have theorized that saturated fats may form "free radicals" (oxidant compounds which can damage normal tissues and even attack DNA) in the blood which aggravates the other factors.

The stressed-out, hurried nature of American meals also may contribute to our heart attack rate. For centuries, "breaking bread together" has been one of the foundations of family, friendship and communal bonding. It is a time to unite against the stresses of the rest of the world.

But in America today, meals have become tools of business -- "power" breakfasts/lunches, "rubber-chicken" dinners. They have fallen victim to the fragmented interests of today's modern one- parent/two-income families.

FACT #3: The French and Mediterranean people eat less fat from red meat since the meat in France is lower in fat and mealtime portions are smaller.

BACKGROUND FACTS: Red meats, especially beef, contain saturated fats (specifically lauric, mystric, palmitic and stearic fatty acids) that promote atherosclerosis and increase the tendency for blood to clot and cause thrombosis.

DISCUSSION: Cheap and available beef has made us a nation of red meat lovers. We often eat half a pound or more at one sitting, and there are still people who lust for a "well-marbled" steak. That marbling is mostly saturated fat and it can act like a stone wall in your coronary arteries.

Ground beef is especially bad; by most state laws, it can contain 25 to 30 percent fat by weight. But since fat has more than twice the calories (9 per gram) than the same weight of protein or carbohydrates (4 per gram), this means that 50 to 60 percent of the calories from that hamburger comes from fat! Nutritionists recommend eating no more than 30 percent (and less if possible) of your calories from fat.

But, you might ask yourself, "If I drink a couple of glasses of beer or wine, I'll protect myself, right?"

LIFESTYLE TIP

Think of red meat as a garnish or a flavoring. Design a meal with a three-ounce serving of red meat as the star but heap the plate with pasta, rice or potatoes and a lot of fresh vegetables. Enjoy your beef, pork or lamb, but select the leanest cuts, trim the fat before preparation and fill up on fruits, veggies, bread and carbohydrates at mealtime.

Research suggests that you will decrease your heart attack risks by 20 to 50 percent over a person who eats exactly the same as you do but who abstains or drinks heavily. **BUT!** You will still face a greater risk than a person who consumes alcohol moderately **and** reduces saturated fat intake.

FACT #4: The French and Mediterranean people eat more of their dairy fat as cheese than as whole milk.

HYPOTHESIS: Cheese butterfat is not as atherosclerotic as the fat in butter and milk.

The French eat about 40 pounds of cheese every year for every man, woman and child; Americans eat only half of that. Dr. Serge Renaud, head of the Lyon unit of INSERM, says that all dairy fat is not equal. His research indicates that in cheese, the calcium binds with the dairy

LIFESTYLE TIP

Even if the fat in cheese is not responsible for promoting heart attacks, it still contains potent high-density fat calories. So, for health reasons, restrict your intake of high-fat cheeses (cheddar, brie) and go for those with less fat (goat, mozzarella).

fat and prevents it from contributing to heart disease. In milk, on the other hand, the fat binds with milk proteins, leaving the fat free to park itself in your arteries.

FACT #5 The southern French and Mediterranean people use olive oil and goose fat for cooking rather than butter or lard.

BACKGROUND FACT: Olive oil is a monounsaturated vegetable oil which contains very little saturated fats and no cholesterol and helps increase the "good" HDL cholesterol in the blood.

BACKGROUND FACT: Goose and duck fat have far less saturated fat than that from most other animals and have at least one half as much monounsaturated fat as olive and other vegetable oils.

DISCUSSION Saturated fats tend to promote the body's production of LDL "bad" cholesterol which leads to hardening of the arteries. Fat from different animals differs widely in degrees of saturation. As you'll learn in greater detail in a later chapter on fats, *saturation* has to do with how loaded the fat molecules are with hydrogen.

Except for tropical oils like coconut and palm, vegetable oils (olive, corn, safflower etc.) tend to be high in polyunsaturated or monounsaturated fats that tend to lower cholesterol. However, even here the playing field isn't level.

Research by Dr. Scott Grundy, M.D., of the University of Texas Health Science Center indicates that diets high in polyunsaturated oils, such as those from corn, safflowers and sunflowers, decreased cholesterol overall -- including the "good" HDL cholesterol. As we'll learn later, the ratio of "bad" LDL to good HDL may be as important to heart health as the overall cholesterol level.

Enter olive oil, the star of the Mediterranean. Olive oil is very high in monounsaturated fat which research has found decreases the bad LDL cholesterol without lowering the good HDL levels.

Research shows that HDL cholesterol can actually scavenge cholesterol deposits from artery walls, which contributes to reversing heart disease.

FACT #6: People in the Mediterranean region lead the world in the regular consumption of moderate amounts of alcohol - - especially red wine -- and particularly at meals.

BACKGROUND FACTS: As you'll learn in following chapters, the regular, moderate consumption of alcohol

- increases good HDL and reduces bad LDL cholesterols,
- decreases the tendency of blood platelets to stick together (aggregation), thus decreasing the chances of blood clot formation and
- decreases clotting by altering the production of fibrinogen, a key clotting protein.

LIFESTYLE TIP

Put olive oil on your bread instead of butter. Set a small container of olive oil on the table so diners can put a bit on their bread plates to dip in. The cookbook section in this book gives some recipes for spicing up the oil.

HYPOTHESES: In addition to those three scientifically proven mechanisms for the protective effects of moderate alcohol consumption, scientists have identified four other possible mechanisms which are backed by existing research, but which need further study before stating conclusively. Scientists believe alcohol:

- reduces the tendency of coronary arteries to constrict during times of stress. This constriction can slow or stop blood flow (especially in an artery already narrowed by atherosclerosis);
- increases coronary artery diameter and blood flow;
- increases the ability of blood to dissolve blood clots that have formed (a process known as fibrinolysis) and

- lowers blood pressure (for moderate consumption only; heavy drinking raises blood pressure).

DISCUSSION: The cardio-protective effects of moderate alcohol consumption have been demonstrated in hundreds of scientific studies and are generally accepted by the medical establishment. That the American people have heard so little about this until recently be because of a large and growing anti-alcohol movement, those who believe that alcohol in any amount is evil and unhealthy.

Medical evidence on alcohol's protective effects has been known at least since the 1920s and has steadily accumulated since then. Unfortunately, a strong and close-minded group both inside and outside the U.S. government has, to a great extent, suppressed information and in some cases has outright lied to the American people about alcohol.

These people believe -- rightly -- that alcohol abuse is a serious problem in the United States and must be addressed. We agree. However, the anti-alcohol coalition is so intent on saving people from abuse that they have left the truth about moderate drinking trampled in the dust.

LIFESTYLE TIP

Grate your own cheese fresh each time you need it; pre-grated cheeses tend to lose their flavors, prompting you to eat more (and more fat) than you would with freshly grated.

Further, in their efforts to help the 7 to 10 percent of the population who are prone to abuse and addiction, they have suppressed information that could help prevent many of the 1,000,000 heart attacks and 500,000 deaths every year. The human suffering from alcohol abuse must be addressed, but so must the death and suffering from coronary artery disease.

You have a right to know the scientific truth even if it runs counter to the "no-use" government policy message. Because alcohol research has been so determinedly kept from the American people, we will spend most of this book discussing the benefits and risks of alcohol.

And now a final word about wine and alcohol before we launch into the details: throughout the rest of this book, we will refer mostly to wine. However, the scientific and medical research differentiating wine, beer and distilled spirits is far from conclusive. Some research indicates that wine may have an edge; other research indicates that beer or liquor may have a slight edge. **At present, there are more studies that lean toward wine, but we don't believe that a firm conclusion can yet be drawn.**

Regardless of the type of beverage, moderate drinkers have fewer heart attacks and live longer than either abstainers or heavy drinkers. New research may find that alcoholic beverages are all equal and that the most important factor lies in the **pattern of consumption**.

LIFESTYLE TIP

To get the most taste from high-fat cheese without busting your fat budget, buy those with the most intense flavors (gorgonzola, romano, parmesan). The more intense the flavor, the less you need (and the less fat you eat) for a satisfying mouthful. Enjoy high-fat cheeses but treat them like red meat; use them in small amounts for flavor and accent.

Medical research shows that alcohol's cardio-protective effect is dose- related. Research on people who tend to abstain during the week and binge on the weekends indicates that, while 14 drinks a week may be protective taken two drinks a day, 14 drinks all on Friday or Saturday night are not.

The trick, then, is not to drink too much; on the other hand, don't drink too little.

Sidebar Four

Wine and Diabetes

Diabetes mellitus is an insidious, chronic disease which results from the body's inability to produce sufficient insulin to metabolize and regulate blood sugar. Untreated, it can cause serious disability and death. People with the condition can suffer from numerous complications including blood vessel damage (resulting in poor circulation which can cause chronic sores and the need for the amputation of toes and feet), nerve damage, increased risk of heart disease, blindness and kidney failure.

Records from ancient Rome show that at least 1,600 years before the advent of insulin therapy, doctors prescribed small amounts of wine to help control diabetes. While physicians of that era may also have prescribed batwings and newt's eye, wine is one ancient treatment that seems to have held up to the scrutiny of modern science.

A study jointly conducted by the University of Pittsburgh's Departments of Epidemiology, Endocrinology, Metabolism, and Nephrology along with the Department of Pediatrics at Children's Hospital and the Department of Surgery at Montefiore Hospital, both of Pittsburgh, found that ***the people least likely to suffer diabetic complications were those who consumed at least one alcoholic drink per week.***

The study, published in the July 1990 issue of *Diabetes Care*, said, "Alcohol is known to induce hypoglycemia [low blood sugar] and has been shown to improve glucose tolerance in both diabetic and nondiabetic subjects, although this is far from a consistent finding ... Other potential benefits might include alcohol's vasodilator, and other cardio-protective effects."

While the Pittsburgh study confirms numerous earlier studies, the authors urge caution because the lower consumption of alcohol among those with complications may be a result of them deliberately restricting intake because of their complications. It's worth noting here that studies showing the cardio-protective benefits of moderate consumption were similarly criticized because critics felt that the control group -- abstainers -- contained a large number of people who abstained because they were in poor health. Subsequent studies found the criticism was unfounded.

Significantly, ***recent research into the mechanisms of the cardio- protective benefits of moderate consumption have shown a possible link to insulin in nondiabetic study subjects.*** A study of more than 1,000 British women, published in the January 1992 issue of the *British Medical Journal*, confirmed the lower heart attack risk among moderate alcohol consumers and noted that those same people had lower peak levels of insulin.

While the body requires sufficient levels of insulin to regulate blood sugar, high peak levels can increase blood fat and cholesterol levels and may play a role in increasing heart attack risk, but the data so far is inconclusive.

It is known, however, that alcohol metabolism does not involve insulin and occurs completely outside the glucose-insulin cycle. Dry table wines, particularly red wines, contain negligible amounts of sugar. However, sweeter wines such as white zinfandel, port and dessert wines, along with most liqueurs and sweet mixers for liquor cocktails have substantial sugar content which must be considered. The carbohydrates in beer must also be factored into a diabetic's insulin-glucose tolerance considerations.

Because treating diabetes is such a vital life-prolonging task, diabetics should always consult with their physicians about alcohol consumption. A little may be good, but you should not make that decision without medical advice.

Sidebar Five

Wine and Gout

The historical treatment of gout usually focused on the Falstaffian consumer of food and drink, paying for the sins of overconsumption with painful attacks involving tender swollen legs and feet.

Today, medical science knows that gout results in a concentration of uric acid crystals in the body tissues, usually those with the worst circulation, like the feet and toes. In people without the metabolic defect that causes gout, uric acid is excreted in the urine.

It is known that heavy drinkers sometimes show elevated uric acid levels in their blood, but this causes no harm unless the drinker's metabolism is predisposed to gout. This may be the reason that heavy drinkers have a higher prevalence of gout than non-drinkers and moderate drinkers.

The heavy drinker has a lot to worry about; gout may be one painful worry, but it's not the one that kills.

To Think About

Research over the past 15 years suggests that the moderate use of alcoholic beverages for institutionalized elders has beneficial psychosocial effects and rarely produces physical difficulties. Wine has enjoyed a certain reputation for facilitating easeful sleep, especially for the old person.— ***Kastenbaum, R., and Mishara, B., Alcohol and Old Age, Grune and Stratton, Inc., 1980, pp. 165-166.***

SEVEN

What's Moderate Consumption?

Almost everyone has an apocryphal story about a friend or relative who has only "one drink a day" which turns out to be a liter of vodka. The definition of a "drink" confounds researchers who conduct epidemiological studies of drinking patterns. These self-reported statistics are usually under-reported although not usually to the same extent as the liter of vodka in the example above.

It's important to recognize that the definition of "moderate" as it relates to your maximum health may be too much for some people.

Research Definitions Of Moderation

Moderate alcohol consumption is that range that maximizes the known cardio-protective and other health benefits without substantially increasing the risk from other factors. Put another way, moderate consumption should be at the level where your risk of dying **from all causes** is at its lowest.

Physicians and medical researchers say that two or three "drinks" per day falls into the moderate category without argument.

A 1991 study done at the Harvard School of Public Health by a team led by Eric Rimm found that people who averaged up to half a drink per day decreased their risk of heart attacks by only 1 percent -- essentially the same as abstainers. From one half to one drinks per day decreased it 21 percent; one to one and a half drinks, decreased risk by 32 percent and those who drank four to five or more drinks per day increased their risk by 50 percent.

> **LIFESTYLE TIP**
>
> ***A generally accepted definition of "moderation" is 25 grams of alcohol per day -- two to three, 4-ounce glasses of wine; two 12-ounce beers and two ounces of 80-proof spirits.***

***"Given that participants in epidemiological studies tend to underestimate their usual amounts of alcohol intake, the actual amounts associated with decreased risk could be somewhat greater."*—Dr. Curtis Ellison, Chief of the Department of Preventive Medicine and Epidemiology at the Boston University School of Medicine.**

But most medical researchers agree that four to five drinks per day push the envelope of moderation into an area where body size and other personal characteristics become more important.

A 1989 study of the relationship of alcohol use and later hospitalization, conducted by the Kaiser Permanente Medical Center in Oakland, Calif., found that of the 82,430 people studied, people who drank more than one but less than three drinks per day spent the least time in the hospital.

The study's authors, Mary Ann Armstrong and Dr. Arthur L. Klatsky, M.D., concluded that, "This study suggests that alcoholic beverage use has little impact on total hospitalization ... In general, the favorable experience of the numerous lighter drinkers balances the unfavorable experience of the heavier drinkers and ex- drinkers."

In this study, heavier drinkers are those who consume more than three drinks per day. Like most studies done in the past five years, this one corrected its data analysis for ex-abusers who no longer drink because of poor health. It also suggested that under-reporting of alcohol consumption by participants could have biased the results.

Dr. Curtis Ellison, Chief of the Department of Preventive Medicine and Epidemiology at the Boston University School of Medicine, wrote in the September 1990 issue of *Epidemiology,* "... given that participants in epidemiological studies tend to underestimate their usual amounts of alcohol intake, the actual amounts associated with decreased risk could be somewhat greater."

Most medical authorities today say that "moderate" consumption lies between one and five drinks per day and that beneficial effects fade rapidly at less than one drink per day.

Several other studies, however, have suggested that the definition of moderate may be higher. The phenomenon of under- reporting may mean that the wide gaps in the definition of moderate are reconcilable.

LIFESTYLE TIP

Based on size differences and body composition, "moderate" drinking for women will be about 25 to 30 percent less than for a man of the same weight.

The key to interpreting this data is trying to standardize the alcohol content of a "drink." While scientists have generally defined a drink as 8 to 10 grams of alcohol, many researchers feel that with the emotional (and often guilt-associated) nature of alcohol, the under-reporting phenomenon affects not only reports of drinking frequency but amounts. For this reason, the drink that people report may be larger and contain substantially more alcohol than the 8 to 10 grams which is recorded by the scientific study.

According to a 1977 article in the *Johns Hopkins Medical Journal*, chronic ill effects are rare below a daily intake of 80 grams of pure alcohol although this amount varies according to the sex, body weight and other individual differences of the consumer. This parallels a statement from the British Royal College of Psychiatrists whose 1976 report, *Alcohol and Alcoholism* estimated the upper limit of moderation as eight drinks per day, now generally accepted as too high.

The Johns Hopkins article, on the other hand, proposed that to qualify as a moderate drinker, a person should consume no more than 0.8 grams of alcohol per kilogram of body weight on any given day and no more than a daily average 0.7 grams per kilogram of body weight in any three-day period.

A kilogram is approximately 2.2 pounds; there are approximately 12 grams of alcohol in 4 ounces of wine, 12 ounces of beer or a mixed drink with 1 ounce of 80-proof distilled spirits. In research circles, 10 to 12 grams of alcohol is considered a "drink."

Let's see what that might mean:

The drink that people report may be larger and contain substantially more alcohol than the 8 to 10 grams which is recorded by the scientific study.

Example 1: A 180-pound man weighs about 82 kilograms; 0.7 times 82 yields 57 grams of alcohol (or 5.75 drinks) as the **upper** limit of daily consumption for this drinker to be considered moderate. Example 2: A 120-pound woman weighs 54.5 kilograms; 0.7 times 54.5 yields about 38 grams of alcohol or just over three drinks per day.

Women have about 10 percent less blood and other fluids than men of the same size, as well as a higher percentage of body weight as fat (25 percent versus 10 percent). Since alcohol does not concentrate in fat, this means that a woman drinking the same amount of alcohol as a man of the same weight, will have a higher blood alcohol concentration than the man.

In addition, one controversial study suggests that women create less of the enzyme that digests alcohol than men of the same weight. But conclusions cannot be made on the basis of a single study.

However, based on size differences and body composition, moderate for women will be about 25 to 30 percent less than for a man of the same size.

It's important to remember that these Johns Hopkins figures should be considered the **upper** limit of moderate consumption; indeed, many authorities would consider this limit as overlapping somewhat with the heavy drinking category.

This range may or may not be too high. On the one hand, most epidemiological studies put the maximum cardio-protection (and minimum cancer and cirrhosis increases) at between one and three drinks per day. However, medical experts have shown that consumption is typically under-reported with the result that the actual optimum health effects may be closer to the Johns Hopkins article than might be apparent on its face.

Some of the best evidence to support this under-reporting hypothesis comes from Rimm's 1991 Harvard study. He studied physicians who, it is assumed, are more aware of scientific methods and the need to report accurately. Rimm's research found that risks of death from heart attacks continued to decrease even when daily consumption exceeded 50 grams per day. Rimm said in a telephone conversation that he believes his reported consumption figures are probably the most accurate of all the epidemiological studies.

Rimm found steady decreases at four or more drinks per day with no sign that heart attack death rates were rising.

Since heavy drinking is known to increase hypertension (high blood pressure) and since hypertension increases the risks of heart disease, the fact that heart attack deaths continued to decrease with consumption of more than 50 grams of alcohol per day tends to support the Johns Hopkins somewhat higher definition of moderation.

Under-reporting may mean we need to re-define moderate drinking.

Most epidemiological studies indicate that the decrease in heart disease deaths starts to level off at about two drinks per day and begins to increase thereafter, eventually catching up and surpassing abstainers. But Rimm found steady decreases at four or more drinks per day with no sign that heart attack death rates were rising.

This is an indication that alcohol consumption in the other studies may have been **under**-reported since they showed cardiac death rates beginning to **increase** at two or three drinks (where death rates in the people Rimm studied were still **decreasing**).

This could mean that in those other studies, a reported two glasses per day might, in reality, reflect the actual consumption of three or four. In other words, people who **said** they were consuming two drinks per day (25 grams) but who were **actually** drinking three or four, artificially biased the results toward the low end of the scale. The J-shaped curve is still valid and doesn't change its shape, but the number of drinks that define each point on the curve may need to be doubled.

If this is true, then the alcohol consumption levels at which cancers and cirrhosis begin to increase may be likewise higher than the earlier

The alcohol consumption levels at which cancers and cirrhosis begin to increase may be likewise higher than the earlier studies indicated.

studies indicated. That means these negative health effects would not begin to show up until consumption was much higher than is now thought. Overall, this would shift the optimum consumption ahead by one or two drinks, putting it somewhere between one and five per day, which is consistent with a large number of medical studies.

But, since Rimm's study, with presumably more accurate subjects included only heart disease and alcohol consumption and did not also study cancer and cirrhosis, this can only be called an hypothesis.

The Johns Hopkins information should be considered an upper limit only -- one which should **not** be approached on a daily basis.

A better rule-of-thumb is the generally accepted, 25 gram (two drink) limit. Indeed, while Rimm did not define moderate in the Harvard study, when asked, he said that 25 grams (two drinks) per day was a "conservative" definition.

While "drinks per day" is the most commonly used indicator to measure health effects, most researchers hypothesize that peak blood alcohol levels may be an even more important indicator of health effects. As you can read in this book's chapter on liver disease and cirrhosis, the liver's inability to metabolize alcohol at a rate that keeps it from accumulating in the blood is reached at a blood alcohol concentration of about 46 mg/dl (.046 BAC).

While still a theory, this could be the line that separates the good health effects from the bad. It would explain why weekend binge drinking patterns (seen in many societies) are less healthy than drinking the same amount of alcohol, but doing it a little each day. This could also answer why wine -- which is most often consumed with meals -- may also be healthier than beer and spirits.

Certainly 0.046 is a good point to stay below: it seems to be the liver's saturation point and it's about half of the 0.08 to 0.10 maximum limits that most states use to determine legal intoxication for drivers.

Certainly 0.046 is a good point to stay below: it seems to be the liver's saturation point and it's about half of the 0.08 to 0.10 maximum limits that most states use to determine legal intoxication for drivers.

The blood alcohol concentration level theory is just that, not proven fact. As you've seen, it has been very hard to conduct accurate epidemiological studies of large numbers of people because of under-reporting and other errors. And while relating health effects to blood alcohol levels would make this much more precise, it is impractical to even consider keeping constant track of peak blood alcohol levels in thousands of people. And to date, no research has been funded -- either by the government, university or private sources -- to investigate this link.

That's why, for your everyday decisions, the 25-gram level (two drink) is so important: the overall body of the best science shows that this level definitely puts you into the lower-cardiac- risk category (even if the under-reporting hypothesis is true) without expanding the limits of moderation.

It's important to note here that many alcohol control advocates who oppose any form of alcohol consumption, frequently distort research data, quote results out of context and rely upon flawed research to support their ideological cause. As stated above (and elsewhere in this book) scientifically valid and intellectually honest conclusions **cannot** be based on a single study. Data must be **considered in the context of the whole body of knowledge** and not taken out of context or over-extrapolated to unsupported conclusions.

This is said to prepare you for alcohol control advocates who will cite pieces of seemingly credible research to "prove" that any alcohol at all is harmful and that alcohol abuse starts at one drink per day. Interestingly enough, almost all of these advocates are **not** M.D.s; a great number of them are social scientists with a poor understanding of medical science and the scientific method. They seem to feel that it's intellectually acceptable to use bits and pieces of research in order to support their social or ideological goals. The overall body of research simply does not support their positions.

> **LIFESTYLE TIP**
>
> ***Drinking patterns are as important as the amounts consumed. While 7 to 14 drinks per week may be moderate, they are im*****moderate -- and unhealthy -- if consumed in a single binge day. The key to healthy, moderate consumption is a regular, one to three drinks per day pattern.**

Significantly, the people behind the **science** of alcohol consumption, who recognize the beneficial effects of moderate alcohol consumption, are mostly physicians and scientists who **are** trained to interpret scientific data. These people are cautious and unemotional, and typically don't project well on television. This may be one good reason why their messages are so often unheard or drowned out in the din of anti-alcohol fervor.

Dr. John P. Callan, M.D., a widely-published Illinois psychiatrist with extensive experience in treating chemical dependency (including alcoholism) writes in the Winter 1992 issue of the journal, *Priorities*: "These NeoProhibitionistic 'drys' are not only generating intemperate propaganda against overindulgence, but also against the publication of healthful effects of moderate drinking. Alcohol has been shown, in reputable scientific studies, to be beneficial for good health. The one-sided attacks should not go unanswered. Legitimate voices should speak out lest unscientific opinion prevail and Prohibition be re-enacted."

What's "Safe?"

"Safe" as applied to alcohol consumption must be defined in relation to: (1) here-and-now and (2) later.

The "later" definition applies to lifetime consumption and drinking patterns. The overall body of scientific research shows that people who are regular, moderate (two drinks per day) consumers of alcohol have an approximately 10 percent lower risk of dying from all causes (and 40 percent less heart attack risk) than either heavy drinkers or abstainers. Put another way: the risk of dying -- period -- is 100 percent for all of us; moderate drinkers delay the inevitable and have a greater likelihood of living longer.

Here-and-now, things are a bit different. **The single most serious result of drinking too much is death** -- most often from automobile accidents. It is unsafe to drive drunk and the safest rule is not to drive at all when you drink.

A driver should **never even approach** the 0.08 to 0.10 blood alcohol concentration (BAC) which determines the levels of legal intoxication or impairment. For long-term health reasons, people should keep their BAC at 0.05 or below and for the purposes of driving, much lower than that. Alcohol's effects vary enormously from one person to another. But in general, people with a BAC of:

- 0.02 to 0.03 begin to experience changes in behavior, coordination and mental acuity;
- 0.05 may begin to feel tranquil or sleepy. The key liver enzyme that metabolizes alcohol becomes saturated at about 0.046. Above this level, BAC will continue to increase; below this level, the liver will keep the BAC from rising;
- 0.05 to 0.15 experience a steady loss of coordination;
- 0.15 to 0.20 are obviously intoxicated and may show signs of delirium;
- 0.30 and 0.40 usually lose consciousness ("pass out");
- 0.40 to 0.50 frequently die when their heart and respiration fail.

Alcoholics and chronic abusers will experience this same progression of symptoms, but usually at much higher BAC levels.

The people behind the science of alcohol consumption, who recognize the beneficial effects of moderate alcohol consumption, are mostly physicians and scientists who are trained to interpret scientific data.

Charts which purport to show "safe" levels for people of various weights are inherently misleading because so many variables affect the intake of alcohol and their effects on a given individual. Most of these charts are based on an "average" 155 pound man and indicate that one drink per hour will keep BAC at a "safe" level. This may or may not be safe depending on the person and the person's sex (ovulation, menstruation and other factors further complicate things for women).

To be absolutely "safe" requires a designated driver or public transport.

Blood alcohol levels can sneak up on people, partly because the pleasure of intoxication make many people ignore alcohol's effects and partly because most people have no way of relating the degree of intoxication they **feel** with the **actual** BAC. What **is** your BAC after a glass of wine; after two glasses? Knowing how **your** body handles alcohol is a vital part of not drinking too much -- both in terms of enhancing long-term health, and preventing short-term tragedies like drunk driving.

What Affects Alcohol Absorption and BAC?

All alcohol is **not** equal.

Some alcoholic beverages are absorbed more quickly than others in ways that can significantly affect how much makes it into your bloodstream and how quickly it gets there.

Some factors are inherent in the drink itself.

- Drinks between 15 and 30 percent alcohol are absorbed most quickly. This includes high-percentage table wines and most dessert wines, ports, madeiras and fortified wines.

- Drinks with more than 30 percent alcohol (60 proof) tend to be somewhat delayed because the high alcohol concentration irritates the stomach lining, producing a protective layer of mucus that delays absorption.
- Some research shows that carbon dioxide content induces the stomach to pass its contents more rapidly on to the intestines (which absorb alcohol more readily). Thus, beer, champagne or drinks with carbonated mixers may cause more rapid intoxication than those of the same alcohol content which lack carbon dioxide.
- Sugar content will slow down absorption.
- Eating food along with alcohol delays absorption.
- High concentrations of non-alcohol organic compounds delay absorption. Wine, especially red wine, is absorbed more slowly than ethanol/water combinations of the same alcohol percentage because of the significant concentrations of hundreds of organic compounds. Likewise, traditionally brewed beer has very high concentrations of proteins, B-vitamins and complex carbohydrates. Unfortunately, in the pursuit of crystal-clear beer, most commercially available brews undergo intensive filtration that removes most of the proteins, vitamins and other organic compounds which are both healthy and retard alcohol absorption. Unmixed distilled spirits are basically water and alcohol with insignificant amounts of other organic compounds.

In addition to absorption factors inherent in the drink itself are myriad human factors that determine blood alcohol concentration. Among them:

- Body mass; the same drink will produce a lower BAC in bigger people than in smaller ones.
- Body fat; alcohol is not absorbed well by fat so a fat person will tend to have a higher BAC for a given consumption level than a lean person of the same weight.
- Sex; in addition to body mass and fat composition, a woman will experience different levels of absorption at different times in her menstrual cycle -- frequently with peaks at ovulation and at the onset of menstruation.
- Food consumption; the more you eat with alcohol, the slower its absorption.
- Illness; diseases can alter alcohol absorption.

- Drugs; many pharmacueticals can alter alcohol metabolism. Tagamet and other ulcer medications can increase BAC rapidly; sedatives combined with alcohol abuse can kill. The effect of illegal drugs can be enhanced by alcohol; this combination can also kill.
- Biorhythms; morning drinking produces a higher peak level of alcohol in the blood, but also disappears faster since the liver metabolizes it more quickly earlier in the day..

To Think About

To help educate people and promote moderation and more responsible consumption, the publishers of this book, Renaissance Publishing, have made a special arrangement with the manufacturers of ENSURE, a microcomputer-controlled personal breath alcohol tester. This small device is about the size of a package of cigarettes and can measure BAC in seconds. Kept in the glove compartment of your car, it can provide a "reality check" for drivers who might be too drunk to drive but unwilling to recognize that fact. ENSURE can also help you relate the physical sensations of alcohol consumption to specific BAC levels, thus helping you to know when to stop. Normally $149, readers of this book can use the postage-paid postcard in the back of this book to purchase ENSURE for just $124. If the card is missing, you can order by calling (800) 845-4671 or (800) 544- 8890.

Sidebar Six

Moderation Checklist

- **Don't feel guilty**. Despite some of the emotional and incorrect information you may have heard, moderate drinking is not only healthy for most people, but also a source of enjoyment
- **Drink moderately.**
- **Don't drink on an empty stomach.**
- **Be aware of how much you're drinking.** The practice of "topping up" a partially full glass can obscure the amount being consumed. The best monitor is to refill only after the glass is empty. Make sure you know how much the glass holds.
- **Pace yourself.** Drink slowly. Sip your beverage; after all the point is enjoyment, not intoxication. If you drink to get drunk, you have an abuse problem. Nibbling on food can help you moderate the alcohol absorption. Another pacing tip is to drink a glass of water or non-alcoholic beverage before refilling your glass.
- **Be a responsible host.** Never serve alcohol without food and plenty of water. Make sure your guests have a choice of appealing non-alcoholic drinks (flavored sparkling waters, fruit juices, fruit juice sparklers, non-alcoholic cider and soft drinks). Be restrained in the enthusiasm of drink refills and topping up. Offer rides (taxi or otherwise) to guests who may have drunk too much.
- **Don't drive drunk.** In fact, don't drink and drive.
- **Don't urge drinks on people who are reluctant.**
- **Beware of straight spirits.** The irritation from the high concentration of alcohol in undiluted liquor is suspected in some cancers and stomach problems such as ulcers.
- **Don't use alcoholic beverages as thirst quenchers.** Your body wants water, not beer or any other kind of alcohol.
- **Don't drink when you're taking medication unless your doctor says it is acceptable.**
- **Remember that *not* drinking is always an option.**

Sidebar Seven

Drunk Driving

The U.S. Department of Justice 1988 study, *Special Report: Drunk Driving*, written and conducted by Lawrence A. Greenfeld of the Bureau of Justice Statistics (report NCJ-109945) concluded that:

- Two percent of those arrested for drunken driving had been drinking wine only; 54 percent had been drinking beer only and 23 percent hard liquor only. Twenty-one percent reported drinking more than one type of alcoholic beverage. If those drinking more than one type of beverage consumed wine in the same proportions as those drinking only one type, this would increase wine's involvement in drunk driving by 0.5 percent (to a total of 2.5 percent).
- Liquor drinkers arrested had a median blood alcohol concentration (BAC) of 0.25; beer drinkers had a BAC of 0.16 and wine drinkers 0.10. Drinkers of more than one type of beverage reported the highest mean BAC of 0.29.

HOW LONG TO WAIT BETWEEN DRINKING AND DRIVING

body weight (lbs)	1 drink	2 drinks	3 drinks	4 drinks	5 drinks	6 drinks
100-119	0 hours	3 hours	3 hours	6 hours	13 hours	16 hours
120-139	0 hours	2 hours	2 hours	5 hours	10 hours	12 hours
140-159	0 hours	2 hours	2 hours	4 hours	8 hours	10 hours
160-179	0 hours	1 hour	1 hour	3 hour	7 hour	9 hour
180-199	0 hours	0 hours	0 hours	2 hours	6 hours	7 hours
200-219	0 hours	0 hours	0 hours	2 hours	5 hours	6 hours
over 220	0 hours	0 hours	0 hours	1 hour	4 hours	6 hours

(The *median* is a number where half the data is higher and half is lower.)

- Of those jailed for drunk driving, 95 percent were male, had a median age of 32 years old, had a racial composition that reflected society as a whole and were more likely to be unemployed and not living with a spouse at the time of arrest.

To Think About

"Italian drinking patterns nicely illustrate the integration of culture, as well as some practical implications of 'the socio-cultural model' as a policy for prevention of alcoholism. In reconciling an exceptionally high rate of per capita consumption and an exceptionally low rate of alcohol-related problems, one notes that children are introduced early to drinking small quantities of watered wine." Agarwal, D., and Goedde, W., Alcoholism: Biomedical and Genetic Aspects. Pergamon Press, New York, 1989, P. 323.

EIGHT

Wine, Beer Or Spirits: Is There A Difference?

Wine, especially red wine, seems to have an edge in reducing moderate drinker's risks of having a heart attack, although the evidence is not yet conclusive.

Even though wine has the advantage in a majority of studies which investigated people's beverage preferences, some research shows no differences in risk reduction among drinkers of wine, beer or spirits. Some key studies have not segregated the cardio- protective effects according to beverage types.

The majority of studies in which the type of alcoholic beverage is consumed was reported indicate that wine is the preferable beverage.

Dr. Curtis Ellison, Chief of the Department of Preventive Medicine and Epidemiology at the Boston University School of Medicine, wrote in the September 1990 issue of *Epidemiology* that "It is still unclear what kind of alcoholic beverage one needs to drink to provide these [beneficial] effects. The majority of studies in which the type of alcoholic beverage is consumed was reported indicate that wine is the preferable beverage, although spirits also produce a reduction in cardiovascular disease rates. Although some studies have demonstrated a protective effect of beer, many have shown it to have a smaller effect on cardiovascular mortality than other alcoholic beverages."

However, data are accumulating from three different types of studies that indicate that wine does, indeed, offer a greater degree of decreased heart attack risk than the other beer or spirits.

A.S. St. Leger and his team at the British Medical Research Council's Epidemiological Unit in Cardiff found, in their studies of factors associated with cardiac mortality in 18 developed countries, "wine appears to account for the entire alcohol effect."

HEART DISEASE RISK

Relative Risk of Coronary Artery Disease Hospitalization According to Beverage Preference

Preference	RR*
Liquor (reference)	1.00
Beer	1.01
Wine	0.89

Source: Klatsky. Amer. Jour. Cardiology. 1986

St. Leger studied the effects of alcohol and fat consumption, cigarette smoking, gross national product, access to health care, population density and many other factors. He found the lowest death rates from Ischemic Heart Disease (IHD) in countries with the highest per capita wine consumption.

"By far the most interesting result to emerge from our analysis was the strong, specific association [decrease] between IHD deaths and alcohol consumption, more particularly with wine. This was not explained away by fat consumption ... or any of the other variables we examined."

Supporting the St. Leger team's results are two studies conducted at the Kaiser Permanente Medical Center in Oakland, Calif. by Dr. Arthur K. Klatsky, M.D., Dr. Gary D. Friedman, M.D., and Mary Ann Armstrong, M.A. One study, published in the Nov. 15, 1990, issue of the *American Journal of Cardiology* indicated that moderate consumers of wine, compared to abstainers, had a 50 percent lower risk of dying of a heart attack and a 20 percent lower risk of dying of all causes. Beer drinkers reduced their heart attack risk by 30 percent and overall death risk by 10 percent. Spirits drinkers, while reducing their heart attack risk by 40 percent, showed the same overall death rate as abstainers.

An earlier study by the same team, published in the Oct. 1, 1986, *American Journal of Cardiology* found the risk of being hospitalized for coronary artery disease was 11 percent lower for wine drinkers than for beer or spirits drinkers.

> ***The risk of being hospitalized for coronary artery disease was 11 percent lower for wine drinkers than for beer or spirits drinkers.***

Even France, which most Americans associate with wine drinking, shows regional differences. The lowest death rate, from all causes, is in the south and in the wine-producing regions where wine consumption is highest. The spirits drinking regions in the west and the beer-drinking regions in the northeast show less cardio-protection and a higher cirrhosis rate.

Why The Difference?

Some studies suggest that wine is more protective because of the way in which it is consumed. "Wine consumption is usually associated with the consumption of food whereas beer and spirits are more likely to be consumed at times other than when food is served," said Dr. Ellison.

Consuming any alcoholic beverage with food, especially meals, will slow down the absorption of alcohol and help prevent the BAC from peaking quickly.

Dr. Ellison has also suggested that of the three types of beverage, wine is the least likely to be used in binges which produce very high blood alcohol levels that are harmful. Other researchers have said that income or other socioeconomic factors may favor wine drinkers.

However, the St. Leger study did not find such linkages. Indeed, studies on rabbits (genetically almost identical and certainly a class-less population) found that, compared with a group fed no alcohol, rabbits consuming red wine had 60 percent fewer atherosclerotic lesions in their coronary arteries. Rabbits (see graph, Chapter 1) consuming white wine had 33 percent less; those consuming pure ethanol and whiskey showed 25 and 16 percent reductions respectively. Those consuming beer had the same number of lesions.

In 1991, two researchers at Cornell University, discovered a compound in wines—especially red wines—that lowers fats and cholesterol in the blood and decreases the tendency of blood platelets to clot.

Therefore, the rabbit study indicates there is a difference among alcoholic beverages; something other than socioeconomic factors is responsible.

"Wines are rich in aromatic compounds and other trace components which give them their distinct character and it may be to them that we should look for the protective effect," said the St. Leger research team.

They may be right. In 1991, two researchers at Cornell University, Evan Siemann and Leroy Creasy, discovered a compound in wines -- especially red wines -- that lowers fats and cholesterol in the blood and decreases the tendency of blood platelets to clot.

The substance, *resveratrol*, is produced naturally by grape vines to protect themselves against fungus attacks. Coincidentally, resveratrol has been identified as an active ingredient in "Kojo-Kon," a Chinese and Japanese folk medicine used to treat atherosclerosis.

Resveratrol is present in grape skins and extracted during the fermentation process. Because red wines are usually fermented in contact with the skins longer than white wines, they tend to have higher levels of resveratrol.

In addition, grapes grown in areas more subject to fungal infection (such as damp regions like France) and those grown organically without artificial fungicides are more likely to have higher levels. The Cornell study also discovered that some winemaking techniques, used to make wine crystal clear, may remove the resveratrol. Unfiltered, unfined wines (an increasingly popular style which leaves a slightly cloudy appearance) may, therefore, have higher resveratrol concentrations.

Creasy cautions against choosing a wine selection based on this first study because they did not have as many different samples of wine as they needed.

He said he has received a number of letters expressing the American "quick-fix" attitude: when, the writers ask, will resveratrol be available in a pill. Probably never. **Creasy -- like most wine/health researchers -- says that wine is to be enjoyed, not taken as medicine.**

Sidebar Eight

"This Wine Contains Sulfites"

Since 1988, all wines bottled and sold in the U.S. must contain a statement the the contents contain sulfites.

Like most cheese, seafood, jams, fruit juice, raisins, dried fruit and many other foods, wine naturally contains sulfites, usually at much lower levels than in these other foods. The government does not require a warning on the other foods, just on wine. Sulfites (usually listed on the other food labels as sulfur dioxide) are added to jams, dried fruits, processed potatoes, some processed vegetables and other foods as a preservative.

The yeasts used to ferment wine produce naturally a small amount of sulfites; sometimes more is added to keep the wine from spoiling, usually in white wines which do not have tannins to help retard spoilage or in lower-alcohol wines. Alcohol also helps prevent spoilage which is why the bottle of brandy that gets pulled out for eggnog every Christmas never goes bad.

Sulfites are harmless for the vast majority of the population -- except for a very small percentage who may suffer an allergic reaction. These people are usually severe asthma sufferers who comprise about 5 percent of asthmatics.

As with other food allergies -- fish, milk etc. -- people who may be susceptible should consult with a physician before consuming **any** food (not just wine) which contains sulfites.

NINE

Reduce Stress; Live Longer and Enjoy It More

Stress is a prime suspect in the things that kill us: heart disease, cancer, accidents, suicide, murder. Sometimes it's acute stress -- anger which leads to murder -- but most often the killer is chronic. Long-term stress leads to the subtle and potentially fatal changes in our bodies that may eventually produce heart disease and even cancer.

Stress reduction is a vital part of good health but an exhaustive treatment of it is outside the scope of this book. What you will find here is food for thought and some tips to get you started.

> ***Long-term stress leads to the subtle and potentially fatal changes in our bodies that may eventually produce heart disease and even cancer.***

Stress Kills

Acute stress can kill, mostly by causing spasms in coronary arteries which can precipitate a heart attack. Acute stress can also kill by dramatically increasing blood pressure. This may cause a rupture of weakened blood vessels in the brain (a hemorrhagic stroke) or an aneurysm in other parts of the body.

It's not uncommon to read of people who died of heart attacks precipitated by bank robberies, earthquakes or other sources of acute stress. But these numbers are miniscule compared to the hundreds of thousands affected by the insidiousness of chronic stress.

Chronic stress increases "bad" LDL cholesterol, depresses "good" HDL cholesterol, makes blood more likely to clot, causes arteries to constrict, increases blood pressure and makes arteries more susceptible to developing atherosclerotic lesions. Chronic stress has been known to depress the immune system, opening the door to many diseases including cancer.

California Pacific Medical Center cardiologist, Dr. Dean Ornish, M.D., has taken the stress connection further than anyone else in the medical field. In his book, *Reversing Heart Disease*, Dr. Ornish says stress may be the most important ultimate cause of heart disease and that other physical manifestations, including high cholesterol and hypertension, may result from stress.

Dr. Ornish's program for reversing heart disease involves stress reduction, a diet drastically low in fat and moderate exercise. He feels that social isolation and the lack of an interpersonal support network are the most damaging factors.

"Anything that promotes a sense of isolation leads to chronic stress and, often, to illnesses like heart disease," Dr. Ornish writes. "Conversely, anything that leads to intimacy and feelings of connection can be healing." His emphasis on meditation and the "touchy-feely" aspects of relationships and human relations have made many traditionalists uncomfortable, but a great deal of scientific research is available to support his contention.

Dr. Ornish points to numerous studies showing that married people live longer than single ones and that people active in a church, club or synagogue have fewer illnesses and lower blood pressure than non-participants. A roommate or even a pet can dramatically influence overall death rates, particularly those from cardiovascular disease.

Research finds the greatest risk of illnesses caused by stress when people feel they have little or no control over their work or personal lives.

Numerous excellent books exist on meditation, stress reduction and developing better interpersonal relationship. Dr. Ornish's book is a good place to start because it integrates these concepts into the framework of better cardiovascular health.

The Mediterranean Family As Cultural Model

The family and societal ties in Mediterranean cultures like Italy, Greece and southern France can teach Americans much about reducing stress through personal connections. Extended families are more common and, as a whole, people are more involved with church and community groups.

The pace is far more relaxed for these cultures. People take more care preparing meals and linger over the eating. There is a

Mediterranean philosophical acceptance that life is fleeting; whatever human wealth and works can be accomplished by driving oneself to the limits of endurance will eventually be irrelevant. There is a very good reason that the concept of *la dolce vita* -- the sweet life -- is Italian.

Acute stress can kill, mostly by causing spasms in coronary arteries which can precipitate a heart attack.

This dilemma was recognized in a letter written to the San Francisco *Chronicle* in 1992.

"Editor -- I am of Irish heritage, and am interested in becoming Italian since Italians seem to have so much more fun (not to mention more sex). If you're brunette and want to be blond, you just go to the drugstore -- easy. But how does one go about changing one's heritage? I know this sounds funny, but I'm serious and would welcome any suggestions your readers might have. I'm sure I'm not the only one with this problem."—Larry McCarthy, San Francisco.

"But I live in America," you say, "and even if my name is Sangiacomo or Orsini, I'm an American and have to live the American pace."

If you accept this premise, then you accept that you have no control over your life -- and that's a fast track to the cardiac unit at your local hospital -- if you live long enough.

Changing Your Life Without Changing Your Heritage

Changing your heritage wouldn't help much anyway. Numerous studies show that "cultural" genetics play little or no role in preventing heart disease. Immigrants begin to adopt American ways of life and eating and quickly lose their cultural advantage. Of course, individual genetics plays a huge role in your health, but the health advantages experienced by ethnic people in other countries is more a function of lifestyle than DNA.

You can make lifestyle changes to decrease stress.

- ♥ Develop family rituals. They can be as simple as hot chocolate and cookies every evening before bed and a set dinner time several nights a week when everyone sits down together without the television.

- ♥ Invite friends and relatives to dinner. Don't make the meal preparation a high-stress event; concentrate on the friendship instead.
- ♥ Stretch out the length of your meal times. One good way to do this is to eat in courses -- don't put everything on one plate. Split your dinner wine into courses too, a little white with salad, a little red (or another white) with the main course.
- ♥ Take a meditation course which teaches you to disconnect from the stress.
- ♥ Watch your body. Research has shown that just as emotions are mirrored in facial expressions and muscle tension, your emotions will respond to facial clues and muscle tension. Smiling even when you're tense or angry will help chase away the bad emotions.
- ♥ Monitor your breathing. When you're tense, you tend to breath rapidly and shallowly. Concentrate on slow, deep breathing and you can break up a bad mood.
- ♥ Relax. Just as stress can tense up muscles, consciously relaxing muscles can reduce emotional stress.
- ♥ Get a massage. Have someone else relax your muscles.
- ♥ Take a nap. Many prominent and successful people take a 15 to 20 minute afternoon nap which reinvigorates them and divides one day into two. If your work schedule is not flexible, take a late lunch and make the first quarter hour a nap.
- ♥ Exercise moderately. Most Mediterranean people avoid health clubs like they do bad fish. But they walk and cycle as part of their everyday lives -- to work, to market, for recreation. Try it.
- ♥ When things are going very, very badly take a quiet moment, relax, control your breathing, smile and visualize an image of some wonderful time in your life. Focus on walking along that beach, catching that fish, gazing on that unforgettable sunset. Transport yourself into the image and out of the stressful situation.
- ♥ Get a good night's sleep.
- ♥ Allow yourself enough time for tasks. Running late causes far more stress than getting up 15 minutes early or leaving for a meeting with time to spare.

- Ask for help. When you're overloaded, rely on friends, family and at work, your co-workers. If you can't depend on these people you need to remove yourself from that situation. Consider professional counseling to help with the motivation and guidance to make this decision and for the support to carry it out.
- Let it all out. But not on your friends. Punch a bag, take a brisk walk where every step is a kick at your nemesis.
- Don't take it out on those who love you.
- If it's been a bad day, take a walk around the block or the yard before you greet your spouse, roommate, children, significant other, mother, father, brother, sister, dog, parakeet. They can't support you if you take your anger out on them.
- Be irresponsible on occasion. You probably have some deadlines, maybe most of them, that won't matter a lot if they aren't met. Don't let your friends or loved ones down, but being a day late on some things won't matter.
- Take a paid vacation day if you're feeling angry, depressed or stressed out. Do something nice for yourself -- go to the beach or the ballpark, get a massage, have a picnic, take a drive. This is a no-obligation, no-guilt, stress-free day for what you want to do, not what you feel you should do.
- If you're single, build your own support relationships by joining a church, synagogue, club, civic group, taking classes, volunteering for charities.
- Get a pet if you're alone.
- Maintain a sense of humor. Read a book of jokes or cartoons; check out a comedy videotape or watch the stand-up comics on television; go to a live comedy club. When you laugh, you're in control and that can keep you out of the hospital.
- Have a glass of wine. Not too many, not too few.

TEN

Cultural Models for Healthy Eating Project

By Greg Drescher

Oldways Preservation and Exchange Trust

As evidence mounts linking diet with disease prevention, Americans are under increasing pressure to change the way we eat. The most recent heart disease and cancer research indicates that we should be eating less food from animal sources. Indeed, colon cancer research conducted for the Harvard School of Public Health suggests that meat consumption should be significantly reduced.

> ***The dominant culinary model in our culture, which puts animal foods at center stage while relegating plant foods to a supporting role (or worse, a garnish), is not contributing to our good health.***

At the same time, all indicators point to enhanced disease prevention through substantially increasing our intake of fruits, vegetables and grains. The broad message is clear: the dominant culinary model in our culture, which puts animal foods at center stage while relegating plant foods to a supporting role (or worse, a garnish), is not contributing to our good health.

Unfortunately, Americans are responding unenthusiastically to the need for more than modest dietary changes. According to recent studies reported in Newsweek, "nearly half of all Americans eat no fruit on a given day and nearly a quarter eat no vegetables. Eleven percent eat neither, and only nine percent of us get the recommended five servings a day." This isn't surprising, as surveys show consumers reluctant to change food selection and cooking practices out of fear that food will no longer taste as good or be as satisfying. Indeed, as Newsweek proclaimed in a cover story devoted to these issues, Americans are "Fed Up!"

Food manufacturers and many in the public health community, apparently believing that Americans are firmly wedded to the culinary model we inherited, are seeking improvement through technology. Some of those strategies are low-fat reformulations of existing food products, the introduction of fake fats and other ersatz foods and the increasing reliance on fiber additives such as oat bran and other supplements. The solution to our diet- linked diseases, this direction suggests, will be found in "techno- food."

Oldways Preservation & Exchange Trust believes there is a far easier, more efficient and ultimately more satisfying approach to dietary change. Look internationally -- and to our own ethnic and immigrant traditions -- for culinary models that combine healthfulness with good taste. From India and China to Latin America and the countries of the Mediterranean, generations of home cooks have developed techniques and recipes to transform fruits, vegetables and grains and small, occasional amounts of meat, fish, poultry and dairy products into satisfying, even spectacular, meals.

Whether the grains are wheat or corn, the vegetables eggplant or bok choy or the flavorings olive oil, chilis, cumin or lemongrass, the collective experience of these traditions proves that diets based largely, but not exclusively, on plant foods can be appealing and delicious.

Indeed, when we confront the embarrassment of culinary riches in these cultural models of healthy eating-models that cast meat and animal fats in a secondary or supporting role, we wonder why so much attention is devoted to techno-food. Or in the words of one French medical researcher, why do we continue to insist on "playing sorcerer's apprentice?"

The conclusion? The widespread existence of healthy eating-models as palatable as the Mediterranean and Asian diets demonstrates that no new food products need to be developed, technologies invented, nor even recipes reformulated to meet the the dietary guidelines. All that is needed is a less myopic perspective on achieving dietary change -- and a sense of culinary adventure.

ELEVEN

Eat Your Fruits and Veggies

The French and Mediterranean dietary customs of:

- eating more fresh fruits and vegetables than Americans and eating them raw or only lightly cooked,
- eating less red meat and eating red meat that is leaner than American meat,
- consuming dairy products in the form of cheese and yoghurt rather than whole milk, and
- eating more grain-based products,

When the data are examined to look at the connection between cheese and heart disease -- there isn't one!

probably account for some of their reduced heart attack rates despite their deadly addiction to tobacco. Many medical experts speculate that if cigarette smoking were eliminated, people in southern France and other Mediterranean countries might have only one-third as many heart attacks as Americans (instead of one-half our rate) and that their cancer rate would plummet.

How does diet influence heart attack risk?

Eating less red meat and eating leaner cuts is a fairly quick way to reduce saturated fat and cholesterol in your diet. Don't give up red meat entirely but limit portions to a three- or four- ounce serving once or twice a week at the most.

The dairy connection is trickier. In epidemiological studies, heart attack rates tend to be very high where the consumption of dairy products is high. But when the data are examined to look at the connection between cheese and heart disease -- there isn't one!

Most cheese is extremely high in saturated fat and cholesterol but it doesn't seem to be as available to the body as the fat and cholesterol in whole milk and cream. Dr. Serge Renaud, director of the Lyon unit

LIFESTYLE TIP

While intensely flavored cheeses like gorgonzola, blue, parmesan, romano and asiago tend to be high in fat, their intense flavor means you can get satisfying flavor without eating a lot of them.

of INSERM, says research indicates that the cheese fermentation process causes the calcium in milk to bind with the fat and cholesterol. The result is that they are excreted rather than absorbed. While the mechanism is disputed by some nutritionists, the "non-relationship" between cheese consumption and cardiovascular disease still exists.

The French eat about 40 pounds of cheese per person each year; Americans eat about 20 pounds. They eat more fresh cheese and less manufactured and processed techno-cheese products such as Velveeta, Cheez Whiz and American cheese (perhaps that last item is a good metaphor for what's gone wrong in our diet as a whole).

Because healthy diets strive to cut down on fats of all sorts, select cheeses with lower fat content such as goat cheese, feta, ricotta and mozzarella. Eat less high-fat cheeses like cheddar and brie.

Your grandmother was right...Now finish your vegetables.

When so many people look to pills and techno-foods for good health, the best advice seems to be what we've really known all along. The old-fashioned admonitions to eat your vegetables and have an apple a day to keep the doctor away may be the best medicine.

Despite decades of resistance from some researchers and important government agencies like the Food and Drug Administration and the National Academy of Sciences (NAS), medical research continues to find that the vitamins, minerals, fiber and trace elements in fruits and vegetables play an important role in protecting you from heart disease and cancer.

Just as today's official government policy belittles the cardio-protective role of moderate alcohol consumption, the "experts" in government have long dismissed the notion that vitamins play a vital role in disease prevention. And just as study after study continues to confirm alcohol's cardio-protective effect, mounting scientific evidence of the role foods play in disease prevention is forcing the scientific establishment to slowly reconsider its positions.

Just as today's official government policy belittles the cardio- protective role of moderate alcohol consumption, the "experts" in government have long dismissed the notion that vitamins play a vital role in disease prevention. Yet, recent research indicates that vitamins may play an important biochemical role in preventing everything from heart disease to cancer and birth defects.

Recent research indicates that vitamins may play an important biochemical role in preventing everything from heart disease to cancer and birth defects. That body of research is no longer being ignored or dismissed as pseudo-science.

"The field [vitamin research] is undergoing a paradigm shift," said Catherine Woteki, director of the food and nutrition board at the NAS in an interview with *Time* magazine. "Paradigm shift" is government-speak for "we're changing our minds and we may have been wrong."

Woteki is co-author of an NAS book which defines (without citing any medical or scientific basis) a "heavy drinker" as anyone who consumes more than one drink per day. Perhaps the NAS will, one day, recognize that the body of scientific evidence on moderate drinking can no longer be ignored and that they will need to shift paradigms again.

Paradigms aside, much of today's controversy rages over whether or not people can get all the vitamins and minerals they need from food or whether supplements are needed for maximum health benefits.

The answer seems to be that both a healthy diet and additional supplements have their own benefits and should be combined. Whole fruits and vegetables contain vitamins and minerals plus both soluble

LIFESTYLE TIP

The wisest course may be to eat as healthy as possible and take supplements for added benefits or to bridge days when eating healthy is not possible.

and insoluble fiber as well as many trace elements and compounds. Science may take decades to identify and then determine their individual roles in health.

On the other hand, considerable scientific research during the past five years indicates a useful role in vitamin and mineral supplements. The wisest course may be to eat as healthy as possible and take supplements for added benefits or to bridge days when eating healthy is not possible. The "health nuts" and "crackpots" once dismissed by the NAS and other establishment organizations may have gotten a jump on good health after all.

What Do Vitamins Do Anyway?

The genesis of both cancer and heart disease may lie in a category of chemical compounds called oxidants. These are produced by the body's metabolism and also are ingested as part of pollution and tobacco smoke and produced by X rays and other radiation, ozone and sunlight. These oxidants are also known as *free radicals* (an organic chemistry term that has nothing to do with a street riot in Berkeley). They attack and *oxidize* your body's tissues, cell membranes and even the DNA that's at the core of your genetic legacy. They may help cause atherosclerosis by attacking the lining of arteries.

Certain vitamins -- most notably E, C and A -- are *anti- oxidants* which help neutralize free radicals before they can do all their damage. Significantly, much of the research has found protective effects at much higher levels than those officially recommended by the federal government and the scientific establishment. For example, the FDA recommends 30 milligrams of Vitamin E each day, but two recent university studies found that men who daily consumed supplements containing 800 milligrams had only half the heart attacks as men who did not.

VITAMIN CHART

VITAMIN	HEALTH EFFECTS	GOOD FOOD SOURCES
C	Anti–oxidant; may reduce risk of cancer of mouth, esophagus, stomach and heart disease; may reduce risk of cataracts; may ease common cold; higher intake associated with higher beneficial HDL cholesterol, prevents scurvy, loose teeth; fights hemorrhage.	Citrus, green/red peppers, strawberry, raw cabbage, green leafy vegetables, canteloup, broccoli, papaya, honey dew melon, kiwi, cauliflower, asparagus, blackberries, raspberries, pineapple, tomatoes.
E	Anti–oxidant; may lower risk of cardiovascular disease,reducing oxidation of harmful LDL cholest–erol inhibiting platelet activity and preventing blood clots; may enhance immune response in elderly; may prevent toxicity of some drugs; may cut risk of cancers and cateracts; helps prevent retrolenta fibroplasia (an eye disorder in premature infants) and anemia.	Wheat germ, oatmeal, peanut butter, peanuts, almonds, brown rice, mayonaise, margarine, corn oil, peanut oil, walnuts, fish–liver oils.
A/Beta Carotene	Anti–oxidant; may lower risk of cancer of lung, stomach, mouth, colon, prostate, breast, cervix; may lower risk of cardiovascular disease; prevents night blindness and xerophthalmia (a common cause of blindness among children in poor countries).	Spinach, carrots, sweet potatoes, kale, winter squash, broccoli, asparagus, brussel sprouts, catealoupe, apricots, liver, egg yolks, whole milk, butter, dark green leafy vegetables, yellow and orange vegetables and fruits.
K	Seems to help maintain bone mass in the elderly, preventing osteoporosis; helps prevent hemorrhage; possible role in cancer prevention.	Leafy vegetables, corn and soybean oils, liver, cereals, dairy products, meats and fruits.
B–6	Appears to enhance immune response in elderly, may alleviate some signs of carpal tunnel syndrome; helps prevent anemia, skin lesions, nerve damage; may protect against neural–tube defects in fetus.	Meat, poultry, fish, fruits, nuts, vegetables, kidney beans, sweet potatoes, rice bran, lentils, fortified cereal.
B–12	Helps prevent pernicious anemia; may protect against heart disease and nerve damage; possibly prevents neural–tube defects in fetus during first six weeks of pregnancy.	Meats, milk products, eggs, liver, fish.
D	Prevents rickets; may help prevent osteoporosis and kidney disease.	Liver, butter, fatty fish, egg yolks, fortified milk. Also produced when skin is exposed to sunlight.
Folic Acid	Helps protect against cervical displasia; may help protect against heart disease, nerve damage, neural–tube defects.	Green leafy vegetables, liver, chick peas, pinto beans.
Niacin	Prevents pellagra; possible cancer inhibitor.	Grains, meats, nuts.

Bruce Ames, a biochemist at University of California at Berkeley, reports that daily doses of at least 250 milligrams of Vitamin C are necessary to prevent oxidative damage to sperm. Ames told *New Scientist* magazine that, "the U.S. recommended daily allowance (RDA) of 60 milligrams per day is too low." Likewise, the U.S. government has no official RDA for beta-carotene despite indications that large doses have been shown to protect against cancer and heart disease.

The U.S. government has no official RDA for beta-carotene despite indications that large doses have been shown to protect against cancer and heart disease.

Of course, high doses of some vitamins can be hazardous. You should restrain the American penchant for believing that if some is good, a lot is better. This is sometimes, but not always, true.

Why Not Just Pop A Pill?

Why would you want to?

Neither wine nor food should be viewed as medicine. They are sources of pleasure which, when used properly, also benefit your health and enrich your life.

Scientists believe that many food components have a cooperative effect which may enhance health benefits that are absent in isolated compounds. This means that it is possible that other, as yet undiscovered or unconfirmed, organic compounds in food may enhance the way that vitamins, minerals and other known beneficial compounds actually work their magic.

We do know that fruits and vegetables contain both soluble and insoluble fiber which play important roles in health. Insoluble fiber provides bulk to speed digesting food through your system. Science believes this increased speed may prevent potential carcinogens from having enough time to cause cancers of the colon and other parts of the gastrointestinal tract.

Insoluble fiber (found in oat bran, beans, the pectin in fruits and many other sources) plays a different role which is still somewhat controversial. One study indicates this form of fiber helps reduce blood fat and cholesterol by simply replacing less- healthy foods. Other studies suggest that soluble fiber compounds actually bind with fat and cholesterol in the digestive tract and prevent them from being absorbed.

Does it really matter to your body how insoluble fiber works so long as eating it enhances your health?

The Question of Garlic

Many studies have indicated that people who eat large amounts of garlic have lower rates of cancer and heart disease. The *Journal of the American Cancer Institute* reported in 1992 on 1,600 people studied in China. Those who ate the most garlic (and related foods like onions, shallots, leeks and chives) had 60 percent fewer cases of stomach cancer than those who ate less.

Many studies have indicated that people who eat large amounts of garlic have lower rates of cancer and heart disease. The Journal of the American Cancer Institute reported in 1992 on 1,600 people studied in China. Those who ate the most garlic (and related foods like onions, shallots, leeks and chives) had 60 percent fewer cases of stomach cancer than those who ate less.

The catch here is the amount you have to eat: 53 pounds per year, about a pound a week. That doesn't seem to bother the average Frenchman or Italian whose recipes so often begin with, "saute the onion and garlic in olive oil...."

A garlic supplement pill, Kwai, is now available.

While supplements may be good insurance, you'll probably find more enjoyment and just as much health in a bowl of pasta primavera (vegetables) with olive oil and garlic, perhaps preceded by an appetizer of baked garlic spread on fresh bread with a thin layer of goat cheese -- all washed down with a glass of wine. Now, that's health food!

TWELVE

Eating Healthy Starts in the Kitchen (Yours!)

Deprivation is not fun. That's why so few people have rushed to embrace the bland, ultra-low-fat, no-meat, self-denial and high-deprivation diets that claim to guarantee you a few extra years of life. That kind of regimen is a Catch- 22: the good news is that you'll live a couple more years; the bad news is that you'll live a couple more years and have to eat like that.

The cuisines of the world provide a myriad of healthy eating models which are delicious and healthy at the same time they are quick, easy and mostly inexpensive.

It takes steely discipline to stay on these diets; they are complicated and time-consuming, which works doubly against their chances of being widely adopted.

Fortunately, the cuisines of the world provide a myriad of healthy eating models which are delicious and healthy at the same time they are quick, easy and mostly inexpensive. Italian, Greek, Provencal, Moroccan, Indian, Chinese and other cuisines have been healthy for centuries -- all without gene-splicing or food preparation facilities that more closely resemble oil refineries than kitchens.

At the end of this chapter is a list of ethnic cookbooks that will give you a start into the cultural cuisines. Remember -- the recipes in these and other cookbooks can usually be made healthier, easier and less fattening by keeping a close eye on ingredients and preparation.

Here are some tips you may find helpful. They are excerpted from *The French Paradox Cookbook* to be published later this year. If you'd like more information about the cookbook, please mail in the postage-paid postcard in the back of this book. If that is missing, write to Renaissance Publishing, 867 W. Napa St., Sonoma, CA 95476 or call, toll-free: (800) 845-4671 or (800) 544-8890.

Tips For Enjoying the World's Cultural Cuisines

(1) AVOID FATS:

High levels of fat, even from olive, ricc or canola oils, are not healthy; you should avoid recipes that call for deep-fat frying. In addition, you can usually cut the recommended amounts of fat in a recipe by one-half or even two- thirds without affecting the recipe. The first time you make a recipe, use one-third less and then work down each time you prepare the dish.

(2) OVEN FRY FOODS INSTEAD:

If you need the taste of fried fish or chicken, try this "oven-fried" technique. Add salt and pepper (to taste) to milk (1 percent fat is good, buttermilk is better) and dip the fish or chicken in it. Roll in bread crumbs until coated and then drizzle with a small amount of oil (1 tsp. or less depending on the size). Bake in your oven at about 450 degrees until browned and crisped; turn the pieces periodically so they cook evenly. Don't broil because that will burn the crust before the insides are done.

Avoid the commercial products that are supposed to do these same things since they tend to contain hydrogenated oils and a plethora of test tube chemicals. Use fruit juices instead of milk and add spices to the bread crumbs for different tastes.

(3) LEARN TO LOVE GARLIC:

Not only is it healthy in its own right, it is used extensively in most ethnic cuisines. To save time, purchase jars of minced garlic preserved with vegetable oil. This is fine in cooked dishes, but crush your own fresh when making salad dressing or garlic bread.

COMPARISON OF DIETARY FATS AND OILS

TYPE	SATURATED FATTY ACIDS (% of total)*	MONOSATURATED FATTY ACIDS (% of total)*	POLYUNSATURATED FATTY ACIDS (% of total)*
Canola Oil	6	62	32
Walnut Oil	9	23	64
Safflower Oil	10	13	77
Sunflower Oil	11	20	69
Corn Oil	13	25	62
Olive Oil	14	77	9
Soybean Oil	15	24	61
Peanut Oil	18	49	33
Rice Oil	17	42	39
Margarine-tub	18	47	31
Cottonseed Oil	27	19	54
Tuna Fat	27	26	21
Chicken Fat	30	45	11
Margarine	31	47	22
Shortening-can	31	51	14
Lard	40	45	11
Mutton Fat	47	41	8
Palm Oil	49	37	9
Beef Fat	50	42	4
Butterfat	62	29	4
Palmkernel oil	81	11	2
Coconut Oil	86	6	2

*Percentages are averaged and thus not toal exactly 100 percent.

Source: U.S. Dept. of Health & Human Services

(4) USE OLIVE OIL INSTEAD OF BUTTER OR MARGARINE:

Use a basting brush to spread a thin layer on bread before toasting and you'll get rich flavor without as many calories as butter or margarine. Use extra virgin olive oil (first cold press) for a nuttier, more intense olive flavor. To save time, and money, combine fresh crushed garlic with olive oil in a small jar to use as a butter or margarine substitute. Refrigerate to keep fresh.

(5) USE CANOLA OR RICE OIL WHEN THE OLIVE TASTE IS NOT DESIRABLE:

These have no taste and are extremely high in monounsaturates.

(6) USE YOUR MICROWAVE:

Microwave ovens are ideal for cooking most vegetables since they steam fast, with little or no water to leach out the vitamins and minerals. When recipes call for sauteing vegetables, parboil them slightly in the microwave first. Then all they need is a quick saute, so you can use less oil without danger of burning. The microwave also makes it possible to use small amounts of butter to flavor relatively large amounts of vegetables, getting that wonderful flavor without overdosing on butterfat.

The Microwave Cookbook by Barbara Kafka (William Morrow, 1987) is a marvelous reference for techniques.

(7) KICK THE SALT:

Highly spiced recipes naturally need less salt. When necessary, use a no-sodium salt substitute like No Salt that works just fine.

(8) USE WHAT'S ON HAND:

Although many recipes call for fresh spices, you can also use dried ones.

(9) EXTRACT ALL THE FLAVOR:

If you've sauteed a piece of fish, meat or poultry in a pan, you can make a tasty sauce removing the meat and adding a half cup of wine to deglaze the hot pan. Reduce the resulting liquid, thicken with arrowroot if necessary, and serve over the meat. This type of sauce can easily substitute for cream-based sauces recommended in some recipes.

(10) SHOP LIKE AN ITALIAN MAMA:

When you shop for food, buy the fresh foods that look best that day and then look for the best recipe. Starting with the recipe first sometimes means settling for mediocre quality.

Shop more often. Huge once-a-week supermarket forays can be an ordeal. Stock up on staples, but buy your fresh food two or three times a week (keeping things simple enough to use the express lane).

Locate a farmer's market; even big cities often have them now. Not only do America's farmers deserve your support but the food is usually fresher.

(11) HAVE THE RIGHT INGREDIENTS ON HAND:

It's frustrating not to have the right stuff in the cabinet. Please refer to the pantry panel that accompanies this chapter for more details.

(12) BUY COOKBOOKS:

A few are recommended at the end of this chapter.

(13) AVOID TECHNO-FOODS :

Pre-mixed foods, as well as many items found in the breakfast food and dairy sections, contain hidden surprises. **Read the ingredients list**. So many foods advertised as "healthy" contain hydrogenated fats and a list of chemicals that defy pronunciation by anyone without a chemical engineering degree. If the product does not list the exact nutritional data (grams of fat, sugar etc.) do not buy the product. This deceptive practice should make you angry enough to swear off products that don't give you enough information to make an informed decision.

If you must indulge, do it with healthy food. The ersatz "shakes" you get at fast food outlets are techno-concoctions with lots of calories. Enjoy those sinful calories by making your own shake from real ice cream and real milk. The same goes for most other laboratory foods.

(14) SERVE BIG PLATES OF FOOD:

Go heavy on vegetables and carbohydrates. Meats seem to get the most care and attention in the typical meal. If you lavish as much attention on the vegetables and carbohydrates, they begin to outshine the animal proteins which means you can serve less meat. This is not only healthier, but kinder on your food budget.

Vary the carbohydrates by exploring rice pilafs, couscous, pasta as a side dish, bulgar dishes like tabbouleh, dumplings or polenta.

(15) GO FOR THE FLAVOR:

While cheeses like Gorgonzola and Parmesan are high in fat, a little imparts a lot of flavor and pleasure. Buy it fresh, not pre-sliced or pre-grated which will start to lose flavor intensity the moment the solid block is broken down.

Experiment with balsamic and flavored vinegars. They seem expensive, but it only takes a little bit; they go a long way. A teaspoon of extra virgin olive oil with balsamic vinegar, fresh garlic and a few spices can be tastier on salads than two or three tablespoons of commercial salad dressing with five times the calorie count.

(16)SERVE FRUIT AND CHEESE FOR DESSERT:

Enjoy lots of fresh fruit and serve a highly-flavored cheese as an accent only.

(17) LOOK FOR SUBSTITUTIONS:

You can find many tasty and healthy alternatives to those "killer" foods.

- ♥ Use olive oil on bread instead of butter; works for most vegetables too.
- ♥ You can substitute two egg whites for one whole egg in many recipes.
- ♥ Many recipes will accept evaporated skim milk instead of cream.
- ♥ Substitute beans or lentils for meat in things like chili, tacos, etc.
- ♥ Substitute chicken for beef.

Suggested Cookbooks

- *Clay Cookery*, Publications International Ltd, 1990
- *The Complete Book of Greek Cooking*, Recipe Club of St. Paul's Greek Orthodox Cathedral, Harper Perennial, 1990
- *Cuisine Rapide*, Pierre Franey & Bryan Miller, Times Books, 1989
- *Southern Italian Cooking*, Jo Bettoja & Jane Garmey, Bantam Books, 1991
- *French Country Cooking*, James Villas, Bantam Books, 1992
- *Verdura*, Viana La Place, William Morrow & Co. Inc., 1991
- *Meditteranean Light*, Martha Rose Shulman, Bantam Books, 1989
- *Cooking Light 1991*, Oxmoor House, 1990
- *Cooking Light 1992*, Oxmoor House, 1991
- *Microwave Gourmet*, Barbara Kafka, William Morrow & Co. Inc., 1987
- *Cucina Rustica*, Viana La Place & Evan Kleiman, William Morrow & Co. Inc., 1990
- *The New Basics Cookbook*, Julie Rosso & Sheila Lukins, Workman Publishing, 1989
- *California Fresh Cookbook*, The Junior League of Oakland East Bay, 1985

Sidebar Nine

A Pantry for Cooking Ethnic Cuisines

The basic pantry for international cooking can be assembled beforehand to save the frustration of missing a key ingredient and the hassle of making a special trip to the store. The following should serve as all around basics to carry you around many of the world's cuisines:

(1) SPICES

- Greek Oregano (mild)
- Mexican Oregano
- anise seed
- crushed red pepper flakes
- cumin
- curry powder
- parsley
- sage
- rosemary
- thyme
- chervil
- basil
- tumeric
- tarragon
- bay leaf
- saffron
- ginger
- chili powder
- whole peppercorns
- fresh and minced garlic

(2) OILS

- Flavorless oils like canola or rice oil
- Flavorful oils like olive, peanut, sesame and walnut
-

(3) VINEGARS

- balsamic vinegar
- red wine vinegar
- white wine vinegar
- fruit-flavored vinegars (raspberry, etc.)

(4) CONDIMENTS

- olives (especially Kalamatas and oil-cured black olives)
- soy sauce
- sun-dried tomatoes
- capers
- chutney
- mustards (Chinese dried, American yellow, French Dijon)
- anchovy paste

(5) CARBOHYDRATES

- pasta of all sorts
- potatoes
- couscous
- bulgar
- rice (Basamati, white, wild, Arborio)
- corn meal (coarse and fine masa flour)
- wheat flour (white, rye and whole wheat)

CARBOHYDRATES (CONT.)

- barley
- Ramen (Asian wheat noodles)

(6) BEANS & LEGUMES

- beans (pinto, navy, black, fava, kidney, cannelli, red)
- lentils
- split pea (green and yellow)
- garbanzos (chick peas)

(7) CANNED & BOTTLED GOODS

- marinated artichoke hearts
- plain canned artichoke hearts
- bamboo shoots
- water chestnuts
- roasted bell peppers
- tomatoes (paste, whole, chopped, Italian-style)
- anchovies
- tuna
- salmon
- white meat chicken

(8) OTHER STAPLES

- sausage, bacon, prosciutto (for flavoring)
- pesto
- fresh herbs
- fresh lemons
- beef and chicken bouillon
- fresh red, white and yellow onions

To Think About

"Wine could increase the absorption of other minerals such as calcium, magnesium, zinc, and phosphorus, as well as iron." McDonald, J., Research Nutritionist, Dept. Health and Human Services, Washington, D.C., Bureau of Foods. From, Wine, Health and Society-Symposium, November 12-14, 1981, sponsored in part by the University of California, San Francisco.

THIRTEEN

The New Temperance Movement And How Your Government Lies to You

In its document, *Healthy People: 2000*, the U.S. Department of Health and Human Services (HHS) set as one of its goals, a 25 percent reduction in American per capita consumption of alcohol. This goal was urged and supported by one of the main anti-alcohol advocacy groups, the Center for Science in the Public Interest (CSPI), a Ralph Nader-sponsored organization. In speeches at numerous public gatherings, HHS and CSPI personnel have said that this reduction is just a beginning and that they would like to come as close as possible to eliminating alcohol consumption in the United States.

The fact that alcohol reduction or prohibition goals have been officially embodied in American public policy -- despite the potential increases in deaths from cardiovascular disease and overall increases in the death rate -- illustrates clearly that the decision-making process rests in the hands of what alcohol abuse expert David J. Pittman calls "The New Temperance Movement."

This parallels exactly the alcohol consumption policies of the United Nations-sponsored World Health Organization (WHO), which predated the U.S. government's by almost a decade.

In the United States, the Surgeon General and the National Institute on Alcohol Abuse and Alcoholism (NIAAA), both part of HHS, are primarily responsible for carrying out these policy decisions.

The fact that alcohol reduction or prohibition goals have been officially embodied in American public policy -- despite the potential increases in deaths from cardiovascular disease and overall increases in the death rate -- illustrates clearly that the decision-making process

Many prominent and respected experts in the alcohol abuse field feel the government's stance is badly flawed.

rests in the hands of what alcohol abuse expert David J. Pittman calls "The New Temperance Movement."

"In 1933, the United States repealed the constitutional amendment that prohibited the manufacture, sales and distribution of alcoholic beverages ... But in the last decade, U.S. society has witnessed the emergence of a new temperance movement which has as its goal the reduction of per capita consumption of alcoholic beverages ... as well as the **prohibition** [emphasis added] of drinking in specific sex, age and status groups as well as in allegedly biologically vulnerable groups" said Pittman, who is a widely published alcohol-abuse researcher in the Sociology Department of Washington University in St. Louis, Mo. His remarks were published along with a series of other papers in *Society, Culture and Drinking Patterns Reexamined*, a book from the Rutgers Center of Alcohol Studies.

Pittman's paper, and others, noted that the federal government and its allied anti-alcohol advocacy groups have targeted for prohibition measures:

- women
- pregnant women
- Native Americans
- African Americans
- the poor and
- the young

The anti-alcohol coalition apparently feels these groups are vulnerable, unable to personally resist abuse or to make valid personal decisions about drinking.

Abuse Treatment Community Divided

Because the government agencies charged with fighting alcohol abuse promote only their official message, the impression is left that alcohol abuse experts are united behind it. In fact, many prominent and respected experts in the alcohol abuse field feel the government's stance is badly flawed.

U.S. government policy is guided by ideology instead of science and prone to distort data to serve an ideological purpose. As a result that policy has contributed very little to reducing abuse.

One of those experts is Yale professor Selden Bacon, regarded as a pioneer in modern studies of alcohol consumption and abuse. He has charged that U.S. government policy is guided by ideology instead of science and prone to distort data to serve an ideological purpose. As a result that policy has contributed very little to reducing abuse.

In a chapter he wrote for the book, *Alcohol: The Development of Sociological Perspectives on Use and Abuse*, Bacon writes: "A great deal of information, 'data,' and communication about alcohol and alcohol 'problems' are available. The largest part of the communication is **noticeably remote from scientifically oriented research** [emphasis added]. Rather studies are usually directed toward proving or disproving this or that particular 'answer,' gaining an ally, condemning an enemy and so on."

Bacon also blasts current alcohol problem researchers because their research "centers on the pathological orientation of studies. They are restricted to consideration of the awful, the strange, the evil, the frightening, the 'sick' or the 'problematic'."

Bacon said later in his chapter, "If astronomers were to limit study to exploding stars or biologists did research only on what were called diseases and freaks, there would presumably be violent critical reaction. The alcohol and drug fields of study need to mature out of their rather primitive orientation to the deviant..."

" In most scientific fields such alleged scientific data* [as used by U.S. government alcohol-control agencies] *would be a, subject for joking. That such so-called data and statistical correlations of combinations of such numbers are taken seriously is striking evidence of the low quality of research in some areas of alcohol studies."—Selden Bacon, Yale professor and alcohol abuse treatement pioneer.

Other abuse treatment experts say that one reason the government funds little research into the "normal" patterns of drinking is because the people who control research grants consider all drinking abnormal.

In addition, Selden says that the current policy behind the alcohol problem movement is "the typical absence of observation of both alcohol 'problems' and of alcohol beverage consumption or consumers. Those authoring such studies rely almost entirely on the records and individual assertions of others, most of whom are not researchers by any stretch of the imagination. Reports of tax receipts or sales are accepted as evidence of consumption in a given population. Records of arrests by police for drunkenness are accepted as evidence of the numbers of persons involved. In most scientific fields such alleged scientific data would be a subject for joking. That such so-called data and statistical correlations of combinations of such numbers are taken seriously is striking evidence of the low quality of research in some areas of alcohol studies."

Money may be one of the prime motivations behind this slanted, non-scientific orientation and many of its incorrect or inflated claims. In a paper published in the November 1989 issue of the *Journal of Alcohol Studies*, Pittman and University of California, Davis professor Dale M. Heien, assert that alcohol control advocates both in and outside the government, "tend to emphasize the extensiveness of a problem in order to attract more attention to their cause. Thus, current economic cost estimates of alcohol abuse can be viewed as one dimension of claims-making activity on the part of the federal government to attract greater attention."

Government and private alcohol control advocates can attract more money and assure their continued employment by distorting data to make the problem look worse than it really is or by ignoring data which does not support their positions.

In other words, government and private alcohol control advocates can attract more money and assure their continued employment by distorting data to make the problem look worse than it really is or by ignoring data which does not support their positions.

One glaring example of such distortions is the estimate of the social costs of alcohol abuse. In its 1990 "Seventh Special Report to Congress on Alcohol and Health," the NIAAA relied on a 1984 study that put the costs at $136.8 billion. In doing so, they ignored a 1990 study conducted for the Federal Alcohol, Drug Abuse and Mental Health Administration which put the figure at $85.8 billion -- about 41 percent lower. The lower estimate came from a study conducted by Dorothy Rice, former Chief of the National Center for Health Statistics.

Despite knowing of the fatal flaws in the NIAAA study (such as assertations that alcohol abusers have per capita incomes more than 10 percent higher than non-abusers or that tuberculosis is **caused by** alcohol) the NIAAA continues to use the incorrect, higher figure.

Bacon commented on this phenomenon, writing that studies like this tend to be "quite fanciful in nature and almost always seem to show close to complete support for whatever program the sponsoring group is favoring."

To build support for its budget and its cause, the NIAAA also uses inflated figures for Fetal Alcohol Syndrome.

As we point out in this book's chapter on FAS, the observed, medically diagnosed incidence of this tragic result of abuse has never been more than one-tenth the rates asserted by NIAAA. To accept the government's estimates would require the assumption that America's physicians mis-diagnose 90 percent of the cases -- a situation which has no valid scientific support.

NIAAA is not always so blatant in using grossly inflated statistics. When faced with irrefutable scientific evidence (such as the scores of studies on the beneficial effects of moderate alcohol consumption) the NIAAA takes a different tack. **The NIAAA ignores the data; uses old, preliminary or unpublished (therefore not peer-reviewed) studies to back up its position and semantically distorts the analysis of the data in order to better support its official policy position.**

> ***"Studies like this* [U.S. government estimates on the monetary cost of alcohol to society] *tend to be "quite fanciful in nature and almost always seem to show close to complete support for whatever program the sponsoring group is favoring."***—Selden Bacon

Government Misinformation

The NIAAA's actions are typical of what Bacon describes as "the 'soft' thinking" so often characteristic of anti- or control or alleviate-alcohol problem movements. This is indicated by behavior and processes such as:

- Describing the whole in terms of only one of the many parts of the whole;
- Allowing metaphors to become descriptions of reality;
- Confusing the ideal or the wish with reality;
- Utilizing one's own movement's propaganda as factual evidence;
- Accepting the proposition that because one thing preceded another, it necessarily was the cause of the other;

- Accepting the assertions of Mr. or Ms. X as an expert in *all* areas of knowledge because he or she was an authority in one such area;
- Asserting that recognizable complex phenomena may be satisfactorily described and fully understood in the terms of one field of expertise and
- Relying upon ignorance, deliberate falsification and manifestly ethnocentric (or other group-centric) thinking."

As with many of the federal government's alcohol-control panels, this one mostly lacks the presence of physicians and true scientists trained to interpret scientific studies and instead is stacked with social science degrees whose training in the rigors of the scientific method and interpreting medical research is not as intensive.

Lies: Subtle and Not So Subtle

Many of the items on Bacon's list of faults can be found in a single document released by the U.S. government in 1992. At the request of the Bureau of Alcohol Tobacco and Firearms (BATF), the National Institute on Alcohol Abuse and Alcoholism (NIAAA) prepared a 34-page evaluation of health claims to provide the BATF a policy foundation on which to base its rejections of any alcohol beverage industry publicity which connected the beneficial health effects of moderate consumption of alcohol. The document was based on reviews of only 23 of the more than 400 responses to the BATF's *Federal Register* notice of March 8, 1991, which sought comment on whether alcohol health warning labels should be amended.

The evaluation of health claims was made by a nine-member panel which included only a single physician. As with many of the federal government's alcohol-control panels, this one mostly lacks the presence of physicians and true scientists trained to interpret scientific studies and instead is stacked with social science or liberak arts degrees whose training in the rigors of the scientific method and interpreting medical research is not as intensive.

As listed in the NIAAA document, the panel consisted of:

- Charles Atkin, Ph.D., Professor of Communications and Telecommunications, Department of Communications, Michigan State University;
- Vicki S. Freimuth, Ph.D., Professor of Communication, Department of Speech Communications, University of Maryland;
- Anthony Garro, Ph.D., Associate Dean of Academic Affairs, New Jersey Medical School, University of Medicine and Dentistry of New Jersey;
- James D. Beard, Ph.D., Professor and Director of Psychiatry, Alcohol Research Center, Memphis Mental Health Institute, University of Tennessee;
- Howard Blane, Ph.D., Research Institute on Alcoholism, Buffalo, N.Y.;
- Nancy Day, Ph.D., Associate Professor of Psychiatry, Epidemiology and Pediatrics, Western Psychiatric Institute and Clinic, University of Pittsburgh;
- Harold Kalant, Ph.D., Professor, Department of Pharmacology, University of Toronto;
- Julie Buring, Ph.D., Associate Professor of Preventive Medicine, Harvard Medical School, and
- Arthur Klatsky, M.D., Chief, Cardiovascular Division, Kaiser Permanente Medical Center, Oakland, Calif.

A spokesman from the NIAAA said that responses from each of the panel members were "synthesized" into the material in the report, but that synthesized material was not resubmitted to panel members.

The NIAAA document analyzed the 23 responses sent to it by BATF and combined them into nine categories for comment:

- Cardiovascular disease
- Moderation
- Fetal Alcohol Syndrome (FAS)
- Cancer
- Unique properties of wine
- New risks
- Specific label messages

- Label design and
- Label effectiveness.

It may be instructive for you to compare the NIAAA's assessments with the corresponding chapters in this book, including the one on evaluating research results.

Cardiovascular Disease

This section* [in the NIAAA report] *referenced only three of the more than 15 studies conducted in 1990 and 1991, all of which confirmed the cardio-protective effects of moderate consumption. This section seemed to imply that the three studies referenced were the only studies on the subject.

Any protective effects from moderate consumption, said this section of the NIAAA document, "has not yet been definitively established." This section referenced only three of the more than 15 studies conducted in 1990 and 1991, all of which confirmed the cardio-protective effects of moderate consumption. This section seemed to imply that the three studies referenced were the only studies on the subject. In addition, most of the referenced studies supporting the viewpoint that more research was needed were much older; many have been disproved by more current research.

For example, this section of the NIAAA report cited the criticism that the abstainer population contains many unhealthy people or former alcoholics who do not drink because of health reasons. NIAAA does cite three studies which have disproved this criticism, but it fails to mention that **every** study since 1988 has corrected for this potential problem and has found the criticism without basis. Despite the body of scientific knowledge, this section treats the criticism as if it were still a valid point of scientific question.

Moderation

Commenting on the benefits of moderate consumption, the paper repeated itself, saying that "potential benefits of alcohol/wine on cardiovascular status have not as yet been definitively established.

Moreover, tradeoffs in terms of potential detrimental effects must be considered in relation to potential benefits."

The preliminary studies it cited in support of this position were all in various alcoholism journals where, as respected alcohol abuse pioneer Selden Bacon points out, the scientific standards tend to be lower than those in respected medical and scientific journals. Responding to industry requests to change warning labels to warn of "excessive" consumption, the report concludes that, "'moderate use may be beneficial to your health' is not correct for all people."

Fetal Alcohol Syndrome (FAS)

The document recommends abstinence for pregnant woman because "it has not been established that **only** excessive amounts of alcohol cause other damage to the fetus."

This section failed to acknowledge the overwhelming body of scientific research which has found no link between moderate alcohol consumption and fetal injury.

> ***This section dismissed as irrelevant the presence of anticancer compounds such as quercetin which is contained in wine.***

Cancer

This section dismissed as irrelevant the presence of anticancer compounds such as quercetin which is contained in wine. While conceding in one part of this section that, "Alcohol has not been proven to be directly, independently carcinogenic for any site," it goes on to state, unequivocally that, "alcohol consumption increases the risk of cancers of the upper alimentary tract and upper respiratory tract." While some research does exist supporting this contention, this section does not mention that many experts and much research exists that emphatically disagrees. This section also doesn't acknowledge that the studies in support of the wine/cancer association have been attacked as sloppy or methodologically flawed.

Unique properties of wine

"There are no specific scientific data to support claims that moderate wine consumption differs from consumption of other alcoholic beverages in terms of potential risks or benefits."

This section does not not mention that, while no conclusive proof exists of any additional benefits of wine over other beverages, most of the studies which have separately studied wine, beer and spirits drinkers have suggested that wine may indeed have unique advantages.

The study group said it could not comment on the assertion that wine was connected with only 2 percent of drunk driving cases because it was unable to locate the study. It took this reporter only two long-distance telephone calls to the Department of Justice in Washington, D.C. to determine that the document in question was the Bureau of Justice Statistics publication "Special Report: Drunk Driving" #NCJ-109945, February, 1988.

***According to Selden Bacon, "Utilizing friends', supporters' and patrons' assertions as independent evidence to support their own programs has been a common practice in the alcohol programs of the past 100 years.* The process takes on rather frightening overtones when government agencies control not only their own action policies, but also the so-called independent research"**

This example was typical of the study as a whole. Research which did not support NIAAA policy was either ignored or, where it fell short in a citation, no effort was made to locate the reference. On the other hand, the report evidenced the panel's energy in searching for citations to support control-group positions, including numerous citations of unpublished, non-peer-reviewed and preliminary work which was accorded the same degree of respect and space in the report as studies which had appeared in reputable medical and scientific journals. Most of these unpublished references were funded by the NIAAA.

According to Selden Bacon, "Utilizing friends', supporters' and patrons' assertions as independent evidence to support their own programs has been a common practice in the alcohol programs of the past 100 years. **The process takes on rather frightening overtones when government agencies control not only their own action policies, but also the so-called independent research**." [emphasis added].

New risks

This section concluded that no new risks from drinking alcoholic beverages had been identified since warning labels went into effect in 1988.

Specific label messages, design & effectiveness

This section concludes that it has no compelling data to recommend changing current warning labels or to add new ones. Having said that, the report devotes five pages of discussion to changing the labels, citing: "NIAAA-funded ... promising but unpublished results ... an unsubmitted manuscript ... quite promising unpublished results," and a Department of Health and Human Services report "advocating" rotating warning labels.

To Think About

"No research has confirmed that an increase in alcoholic beverage taxes would be an effective tool against alcohol abuse. To the contrary, indexing prices of alcoholic beverages so that they maintain a steady relationship to prices of other goods during inflation assumes price elasticity that has been disproven among heavy drinkers in many societies." Heath, D.B., "Environmental Factors in Alcohol Use and Its Outcomes," Alcoholism: Biomedical and Genetic Aspects. edts. Goedde, HW and Agarwal DP, Pergamon Press, New York, 1989, p. 316.

Sidebar Ten

Some Major Goals of The New Temperance Movement

From: "The New Temperance Movement," by David J. Pittman, published in *Society, Culture and Drinking Patterns Reexamined,* by the Rutgers Center of Alcohol Studies, 1992.

To support the U.S. government's goal of reducing American per capita alcohol consumption 25 percent by the year 2000, Pittman's published work lists the following goals:

- ♥ Restricting advertising, including a ban on ads in both print and electronic media;
- ♥ Eliminating business tax deductions for alcoholic beverage ads;
- ♥ Mandatory health warnings on alcoholic beverage containers. (Already enacted into law; proponents are now asking for stronger warnings.}
- ♥ Raising the minimum drinking age to 21. (Already enacted into law. A recent university study found that this measure has **not** decreased teenage drunk driving);
- ♥ Increasing taxes on alcoholic beverages. (Federal tax increase in 1991; many states have increased or are considering increases);
- ♥ Earmarking alcoholic beverage taxes to defray costs of abuse programs.
- ♥ Restricting alcoholic beverage sales by: decreasing the number of stores, bars and restaurants which can sell it, limiting the days and hours of sales and limiting the number of sales outlets in lower-income communities. (Some restrictions have been enacted in local communities including areas of San Diego, Calif.);
- ♥ Legislative price controls on alcoholic beverages;
- ♥ Mandatory alcohol industry funding of public service advertisements to point out the social and health damage of alcoholic beverages and,
- ♥ Requiring ingredient labeling (currently being considered by the U.S. Bureau of Alcohol, Tobacco and Firearms).

FOURTEEN

The Good, The Bad and The Drugly

By Wells Shoemaker M.D.

Don't Do Drugs. We Can Wait.

—Mortuary Billboard in Bakersfield, Calif.

Alcohol and Other Drugs

—U.S. Office of Substance Abuse Prevention

Religion is the Opium of the People

—Karl Marx

Just Say No

—Nancy Reagan

Drug! This four-letter word has recently joined our country's growing lexicon of guttural expletives for wartime enemies: Rebs, Japs, Krauts, Reds, Gooks.

Drug stores have disappeared from America's Chambers of Commerce. We now have pharmacies.

Drugs have been used by cultures of the world since before the dawn of recorded history. The use of mind altering drugs and the criminal culture associated with the sale of illegal drugs has turned the very word into a one-syllable emotional dagger, a rallying cry for Americans. We now have a Drug War.

What is a "drug" that earns such reflexive loathing? In cold pharmacological terms, a drug is a substance -- a molecule -- which has an effect upon the human body's function.

Are drugs inherently good or bad?

There are both medical and social answers, which hinge upon the questions:

- What does it do?
- How much does one use?
- Why does one use it?
- Who decides?

Let's look at what each of these things can mean.

What it does. Some drugs have such one-sided properties that good versus bad seems obvious. The poisonous alkaloid from *Amanita phalloides* mushrooms kills a man in gruesome fashion, while the bitter extract from *Cinchona* bark (quinine) cures malaria.

How much. Many drugs can be either helpful or harmful depending upon dosage. The extract from foxglove leaves, *digitalis*, can be lifesaving in proper dosage but lethal in overdose. Conversely, *botulinus* toxin is a ferocious poison in the amounts found in poorly preserved canned goods, yet quite useful therapeutically when diluted and used to relieve muscle tremors.

Why one uses it. Hallucinogenic mescaline from *peyote* cactus has served as part of a traditional, centuries old, religious ritual in Native American cultures. However, when sold to students on the streets of a modern city, the same substance becomes a criminal commodity. Cocaine was the first medically effective local anesthetic, and it remains a valuable drug for ear, nose, and throat surgery. Yet, obviously, it is a dangerous and addictive drug when used to get high. Human intention, rather than biochemical properties, define good versus bad in these examples.

Who decides. Society's values clearly may dictate whether a drug is good or bad. Wine, for example, is an integral part of religious rituals in both the Jewish and the Catholic faiths. Is the alcohol in wine a "drug" when used in communion, or a sacred symbol? Sociologists might debate, but there would be no debate from an Islamic fundamentalist, for whom the very same glass of wine would be a despicable evil, a sinful indulgence.

Organic Drugs?

The purification, concentration, or synthetic alteration of natural drugs tends to increase the potency and specificity of the drugs.

Most drugs in the world occur naturally and just happen to affect people. The drug effects upon humans, whether good or bad, generally have little to do with the natural functions of the molecules in the living organisms that made them.

The sticky resin from the damaged seed pod of a red poppy relieves pain, induces sleep, and causes constipation in humans. *Resveratrol*, a natural phenolic compound found in grape skins, protects against fungal attack on the grapes, but coincidentally lowers cholesterol in people.

Taxol from the bark of the Pacific yew combats cancer of the ovary and breast. *Quercetin*, found in several vegetables as well as grape wine, has anti-cancer properties in mammals.

People who eat bread made from spoiled grain may suffer excruciating pain, delirium, and death from *ergot* poisoning. Pharmaceutical amounts of ergot alkaloids can relieve migraine headaches and stanch hemorrhage after childbirth. *Aflatoxin*, produced by a different fungus in moldy grain, causes cirrhosis of the liver. Ethanol, produced by yeast as bread rises or as grapes ferment, dilates blood vessels. Presumably, these effects are not prime concerns of the fungi that made the drugs.

Better Living Through Chemistry?

The purification, concentration, or synthetic alteration of natural drugs tends to increase the potency and specificity of the drugs. For example, plain penicillin, a drug produced by a greenish mold, kills the strep bacteria that cause scarlet fever. Chemical modification of penicillin has created antibiotics that kill a much broader variety of disease-causing germs.

Morphine is a more potent analgesic than the crude opium from which it is extracted. Synthetic heroin is more powerful still, both in its pain-relieving effects and its toxic side effects in overdosage. Coca

Distillation of wine or beer to produce more concentrated ethanol solutions led Thomas Jefferson to coin the term "ardent spirits." He also identified them as more harmful to both the individual and society than wine.

leaves have long been chewed safely by native Andeans, but purified cocaine powder can cause fatal cardiac standstill, seizures, and strokes in healthy young adults.

Distillation of wine or beer to produce more concentrated ethanol solutions led Thomas Jefferson to coin the term "ardent spirits." He also identified them as more harmful to both the individual and society than wine.

In general, the use of purified or synthetic drugs in abusive fashion leads to more dramatic -- and more dangerous -- effects than the "natural" ones.

Abuse and Addiction

Drugs of abuse are biologically active substances taken **intentionally** and **voluntarily** by individuals **contrary to the prevalent values of society**. Recalling that these values may differ radically between cultures of the world and epochs of history, we must still ask: "Why would someone abuse drugs and risk both society's disapproval and physical dangers?"

Stated bluntly, drugs of abuse do something that the user *likes*. Usually this effect involves alteration of state of mind, often a retreat from the reality of grim circumstances. "Recreational" users take drugs just to have fun or to heighten sexual experiences.

One of the best advertised consequences of drug abuse is **addiction**. Like "allergy", "addiction" tends to be a widely misused word. A strict medical definition includes several elements:

- Tolerance. An addicted individual can use progressively more of a substance before achieving the desired drug effect.
- Physical dependence. Withdrawal of the substance causes adverse symptoms that can be avoided by continued use of the drug.

- Psychological attachment. An individual develops a craving for the substance, often compulsively searching out and using the substance despite overtly negative physical, emotional, and social consequences. Denial of this dependence characterizes nearly every addicted individual.

Is alcohol a "drug?" Surely, yes, without a doubt. Alcohol is a natural, organic substance that has an effect upon the human body. But...is it a "good" drug or a "bad" drug? The answer depends upon the response to the four questions defined earlier.

The War and the Crimes

If society, or one of its respected agents (a doctor), offers a patient a release from painful or desperate straits, society defines the action as humane, compassionate, or therapeutic. In Aldous Huxley's *Brave New World,* the government of a fictional futuristic society dosed its citizens with "soma" to keep them submissively content.

However, if an individual chooses to dose himself on his own, without permission from society, then the drug use becomes "bad" and usually illegal. Users become outlaws, but the damage doesn't stop there.

The lack of product integrity of illegal drugs poses a lethal threat: unreliable potency, adulterated drugs, and toxic contaminants; all can kill or disable even casual drug users. Deprived of technological advances in packaging and sterility, abusers of injected drugs face mortal health threats from infection.

While the isolation, alienation, lost productivity, and poor health of drug abusers causes predictable personal and family stress, there is a far more socially corrosive consequence of drug abuse. The criminal behavior attached to the sale and distribution of illegal drugs adds a destructive dimension that touches every corner of American life. Drug users steal relentlessly to pay the inflated prices for their drugs. Dealers kill other dealers to secure the franchise of selling.

If alcohol is used to blot out an unhappy experience or cope with a sense of failure or despair, then this is a "bad" drug.

Children, policemen, health institutions, schools, and maybe our national conscience, are caught in a merciless crossfire of economic privation, social decay, and lead bullets.

In the Prohibition era of the 1920s, alcohol was the focus of this fusillade. Now the production and sale of alcohol is legal. It's also possibly the most meticulously regulated, crime-free activity in the U.S.A. The firing continues on the front of the "other drugs."

Alcohol and Other Drugs?

Is alcohol a "drug?" Surely, yes, without a doubt. Alcohol is a natural, organic substance that has an effect upon the human body. But...is it a "good" drug or a "bad" drug? The answer depends upon the response to the four questions defined earlier.

1. What does it do?

Alcohol affects mental functions, coordination, blood vessel tone, and urinary concentration, to name a few. It also raises HDL cholesterol and decreases the tendency for clots to form in arteries.

2. How much do you use?

Clearly, *excessive* use of alcohol can cause clumsiness, poor judgment, and poor impulse control. Prolonged heavy use can cause liver disease and heart muscle disorders and may contribute to throat cancer.

Moderate use, on the other hand, causes no measurable increase in chronic disease. In fact, moderate use affords its users a 20 to 40 percent reduction in the risk of heart attacks and a reduction in mortality from all causes, when compared to the extremes of both abstention and abuse.

3. Why do you use it?

If alcohol is used to blot out an unhappy experience or cope with a sense of failure or despair, then this is a "bad" drug. *It doesn't work.* If served to a naive teenager far from the safety and guidance of home, or if served to a drunken man about to drive a car, then this is a "bad" drug. *It's dangerous.* If consumed in large quantities by a pregnant woman, then this is a "bad" drug. **It causes birth defects** in heavy dosage.

If wine is served in moderation with a family meal, admired for its color and aroma, valued for its flavor, and esteemed for the years of skill required to make it, wine is more aptly considered a food than a drug.

If wine is served in moderation with a family meal, admired for its color and aroma, valued for its flavor, and esteemed for the years of skill required to make it, wine is more aptly considered a food than a drug. If served to brighten the pleasure of a meal for a person on a low salt diet, wine is a food. If wheedled to call it a drug because it contains alcohol, and then obliged to label it "good" or "bad," I would say, "Good," with conviction.

4. Who Decides?

Alcohol in the form of wine on the dinner table in Italy is an honored national custom. In Bagdad, it's a felony. On the altar, it's a communion with God. In high school, it's a felony.

A New Prohibition Era?

Alcohol, like many substances we use or consume daily, is a drug -- one capable of both beneficial and detrimental effects, one with complex interactions with an individual, family, and society.

One-issue alcohol antagonists depict alcohol in any form as a "drug" in its most toxic and vile connotation. Intelligent, community-minded people who enjoy wine -- or make it -- are denigrated with the same tarry brush as crazed, ruthless, drug- dealing gangs. This is an incorrect and simplistic tactic.

The anti-alcohol groups deprecate and suppress medical facts that have clear relevance to a nation that loses half a million citizens a year to heart disease, while exaggerating the value of studies supporting their viewpoint. They tell lies in public about issues of great sensitivity, such as the threat to the fetus from a mother's light drinking.

The question, *"Who Decides?"* reverberates as anti-alcohol groups talk about "Alcohol and Other Drugs." These people ignore such fundamentally crucial issues as dosage and lumping moderate use and abuse as extensions of the same dangerous habit. They ignore centuries of cultural experience and millennia of religious precedent.

The anti-alcohol groups deprecate and suppress medical facts that have clear relevance to a nation that loses half a million citizens a year to heart disease, while exaggerating the value of studies supporting their viewpoint. They tell lies in public about issues of great sensitivity, such as the threat to the fetus from a mother's light drinking, as though Americans cannot be trusted to handle balanced information.

Conclusion—Just Say Know.

People can be trusted with both the truth and the humble uncertainties of science. No sane person disputes the potential of alcohol, when abused, to cause harm.

Rather than seeking bumper-sticker solutions, our country needs to develop a culture of responsible decision-making by both our youth and our mature citizens.

Americans need to support medical research to understand the causes and medical therapy to relieve the burdens caused by the abuse of alcohol, while preserving the ability of moderate people to use this "drug" in a pleasurable, healthful, and legal fashion.

FIFTEEN

Alcohol Abuse: Defining It, Avoiding It

There is no doubt that alcohol can be a two-edged sword: while moderation can make the overwhelming majority of us healthier, heavy drinking and abuse has the potential to cause ill health, misery and death for an estimated seven to ten percent of the American population.

People who abuse alcohol, according to substance abuse experts, usually have problems controlling other compulsive behavior.

This is a very complex problem about which hundreds of books and scholarly articles have been written. Any treatment of this subject in a book such as this risks over-simplifying the problem; despite this risk, this is a subject that needs to be raised even though space here does not allow an exhaustive treatment.

Alcohol abuse, alcoholism, problem drinking, dependency: whatever it's called it should not be minimized. Everyone, not just alcohol consumers, should be aware of the signs of abuse and dependency. We should take quick, early action to stop drinking or seek treatment (or to urge a friend or loved one to stop or seek help) if drinking exceeds moderation.

People who abuse alcohol, according to substance abuse experts, usually have problems controlling other compulsive behavior. These people are often abusers of other substances -- almost always tobacco -- and frequently cocaine and other illegal drugs as well as tranquilizers and other prescription drugs. They also tend to have other compulsive disorders associated with food (obesity or anorexia) or behavior.

Defining Abuse

One of the most commonly used devices to help detect current or potential alcohol problems is the Michigan Alcohol Screening Test (MAST). A score of 5 or more on the test is considered an indication of dependency. Among many questions, the test asks if the person being tested:

- Has ever been arrested for drunken driving (yes = 2 points).
- Has ever gotten into trouble at work because of drinking (yes = 2 points).
- Has ever neglected personal obligations (work or family) because they were drinking (yes = 2 points).
- Has ever been in a hospital because of drinking (yes = 5 points).
- Has ever been to anyone for help with drinking (yes = 5 points).

The test also asks the person if:

- They feel they are a normal drinker (no = 2 points).
- Their friends or relatives think they are normal drinkers (no = 2 points).

The MAST test aims at detecting more full-blown cases of alcohol abuse. Experts say that detecting a developing dependency is far more important to the individual because it is easier to treat the earlier it is detected.

Heavy drinking is usually one of the first signals. Although some people may develop a psychological dependence on one or two glasses per day, this is not common. The scientific definitions of moderate versus heavy drinking are discussed at length in this book's chapter on moderation. In general, however, the broad mass of scientific research defines moderate as 25 grams of alcohol per day (two to three drinks) and heavy drinking at about 50 grams per day or more.

Other signs which may be a warning of alcohol abuse include:

- Orienting personal activities around drinking;
- Drinking at the same time each day;
- The inability to have fun without drinking;
- Drinking for courage or to relieve sadness or depression;

- Increased tolerance for alcohol (that is, it takes more alcohol to get intoxicated);
- Frequent absences from work or family obligations due to drinking and
- Physical withdrawal symptoms in the absence of alcohol such as nausea, nervousness, lack of concentration, sweating.

It's important to note that the the definition of heavy drinking and abuse have been blurred in recent years by anti-alcohol advocates who have consistently attempted to redefine "heavy" drinking as more than three to four glasses per week. Most substance abuse experts say this attempt to make the glass-of-wine-per-day sipper a "heavy drinker" devalues the impact of true abuse and, in the process, hinders their ability to treat those people who are truly alcoholics.

The definition of heavy drinking is driven by the economic concerns of hospitals and clinics who have found substance abuse a very profitable medical practice and an efficient way to fill empty beds. Most substance abuse experts say this attempt to make the glass-of-wine-per-day sipper a "heavy drinker" devalues the impact of true abuse and, in the process, hinders their ability to treat those people who are truly alcoholics.

Many health industry experts say that this "ratcheting down" of the definition of heavy drinking is driven by the economic concerns of hospitals and clinics who have found substance abuse a very profitable medical practice and an efficient way to fill empty beds. It is in the economic self-interest of those in the alcohol treatment industry to diagnose as heavy drinkers people who are actually consuming moderate and healthy amounts of alcohol. The abuse treatment industry has an audience for its advertising and promotional efforts if, as some people assert, **any** amount of alcohol consumption is bad and unhealthy.

Who Is at Special Risk From Alcohol Consumption?

Some people should be especially careful when considering their choice to consume alcoholic beverages. They include:

It is in the economic self-interest of those in the alcohol treatment industry to diagnose as heavy drinkers people who are actually consuming moderate and healthy amounts of alcohol.

- The 7 to 10 percent of Americans who have compulsive disorders that make it impossible to consume moderately;
- People suffering from mental illnesses, particularly manic depression;
- People with hypertension, gout, ulcers or diabetes. Alcohol consumption does not cause these disorders, but heavy drinking can aggravate them. Moderate drinking **with your doctor's consent**, however, can have beneficial effects on diabetes and possibly hypertension;
- Women, who are usually smaller and have less body fluids than men of the same size, resulting in higher blood alcohol concentration from the same amount of alcohol consumed;
- Pregnant women, although a consistent body of more than two dozen studies have failed to find any association between up to 10 drinks per week and any effect on the developing fetus;
- Women with a history of breast cancer in their immediate relatives (sisters, mothers) and
- Men whose wives or significant others are trying to conceive.

Avoiding Abuse

While abstinence may seem like the best way to prevent abuse, experiments with prohibition in America and draconian control in Europe show this is not practical. What's more, the scientifically proven connection between alcohol and beneficial health effects for most people show that abstinence is not always desirable.

Given all that, the important personal health issue is to determine what puts people at greater risk of abuse, and then decide how to reduce or eliminate that risk.

Alcohol abuse seems to have some genetic connection. Studies on twins have shown that it's more likely that identical twins will abuse alcohol than will fraternal twins. Likewise, family studies have shown that children of abusers are more likely to be abusers themselves. Some genetic predisposition is undoubtedly at work in both cases, but most studies show that family behavior and what children learn in the home is far more important.

A number of studies have shown that families in which one parent was an alcoholic, but which continue to carry on with rituals, such as regular dinner times and holiday celebrations, produce fewer alcoholic children in later life.

A study conducted by psychiatrist Dr. Stephen Wolin, M.D., at George Washington University and anthropologist Linda Bennett at Memphis State University studied 68 married men and women who had an alcoholic parent. Of the 31 whose parents were least deliberate at carrying on family rituals, there were 24 alcoholics. But among the 12 whose parents were the **most deliberate** at maintaining family rituals, there were only 3 alcoholics.

Indeed, the study also found a markedly reduced incidence of abuse among children of alcoholics who married people coming from families with strong rituals.

Societal rituals, practices and expectations also exert enormous influence over drinking and help promote or control abuse. The Mediterranean model of alcohol consumption, where alcohol is freely available and consumed but which has relatively little alcoholism contrasts with northern Europe and America where alcohol consumption is strictly controlled (by guilt, religion and government), consumed in smaller amounts and where alcoholism is a far greater problem.

Societal rituals, practices and expectations also exert enormous influence over drinking and help promote or control abuse. The Mediterranean model of alcohol consumption, where alcohol is freely available and consumed but which has relatively little alcoholism contrasts with northern Europe and America where alcohol

World Health Organization (WHO), Italy, which makes more wine than any other country in the world and has the second highest wine consumption in the world (approximately 19 gallons per person per year), has less than one-seventh the rate of alcoholism (500 per 100,000) as the United States (3,750 per 100,000) which drinks only about one half gallon of wine per person per year.

consumption is strictly controlled (by guilt, religion and government), consumed in smaller amounts and where alcoholism is a far greater problem.

According to the U.N.'s World Health Organization (WHO), Italy, which makes more wine than any other country in the world and has the second highest wine consumption in the world (approximately 19 gallons per person per year), has less than one-seventh the rate of alcoholism (500 per 100,000) as the United States (3,750 per 100,000) which drinks only about one half gallon of wine per person per year.

Wine is a key part of this equation since it is the beverage most often consumed moderately and with food. Bingers most often use beer and spirits. In fact, in one key indicator of the tragic consequences of alcohol abuse -- drunk-driving accidents -- the U.S. Department of Transportation reported that wine was a factor in only 2 percent of the incidents.

In Italy and Greece, wine is consumed in small amounts and almost always with food. People who drink too much are social outcasts. Wine in these cultures is simply another food to be enjoyed and is notable by its lack of specialness. Unfortunately, many northern European habits are working their ways south, among them a shift to liquor and beer which are drunk mostly by themselves, especially by young "hip" Italians. This has resulted in an unfortunate increase in alcoholism and alcohol-related traffic accidents.

In one key indicator of the tragic consequences of alcohol abuse -- drunk-driving accidents -- the U.S. Department of Transportation reported that wine was a factor in only 2 percent of the incidents.

By contrast, in northern Europe, especially in the Scandinavian countries, alcohol is heavily regulated, punitively taxed and imbued with great moral significance. The relatively rare state-controlled alcohol stores in Finland and Sweden are sterile and unappealing by American standards; advertising is not allowed and taxes are double or triple those in other European countries. In Sweden, each community has a Temperance Board to which people who may have a drinking problem are referred. Despite the best intentions of these liberal countries' social engineers, public drunkenness and binge drinking is common. In Finland, strict sales and advertising controls on alcohol, and a national Department of Sobriety, along with moral approbation for almost any level of consumption, have produced:

- A Finnish rate of arrests for drunkenness of about 7 percent of the population, higher than any other European country;
- Government estimates that Finns consume more illegally brewed alcohol than is bought in stores and
- A death rate from acute alcohol poisoning that is about five times higher than Denmark which, alone of the Scandinavian countries, lacks draconian alcohol control laws.

To their credit, however, the Scandinavian countries have reduced drunk-driving accidents to approximately 10 percent of driving accidents, as opposed to the estimated 25 to 50 percent in the U.S. Research shows that this is partly due to strict penalties for drunk driving, but mostly because of efficient and extensive public transportation which reduces the reliance on automobiles.

So it seems that, in addition to cutting heart attack risks in half and decreasing the overall death rate by more than 10 percent, moderate consumption of alcohol, especially wine, with meals is an effective way to reduce the risk of abuse -- except for the 7 to 10 percent of Americans who cannot consume it moderately and for whom abstinence seems to be the best option. But since research indicates that taxation, availability control and moral prohibitions do not work, and, further, that much of the abuse seems to be learned rather than inherited, the best protection of all against abuse may be:

- ♥ a moderation mindset, combined with
- ♥ education and
- ♥ a coherent family with strong rituals.

To Think About

"The evidence is that control-of-supply policies will never reduce substance abuse significantly and that such policies may backfire by propagating images of substances as being inherently overpowering." —Peele, S., "The Limitations of Control-of-Supply Models for Explaining and Preventing Alcoholism and Drug Addiction." Journal of Studies and Alcohol, Vol. 48, No. 1, p. 61, 1987.

SIXTEEN

Evaluating Risks And Benefits:

Aspirin And Alcohol

If medical science came up with a miracle drug that could cut America's leading cause of death -- fatal heart attacks -- almost in half, people would rush to the drugstore for a dose of this lifesaving pharmacuetical. This happened.

The year was 1989; the miracle drug was aspirin. Yet another lifesaver, moderate alcohol consumption, has the potential to save **many more lives than aspirin**, and has been ignored and abused by the American government.

Yet another lifesaver, moderate alcohol consumption, has the potential to save many more lives than aspirin, and has been ignored and abused by the American government.

Comparing the health effects of aspirin and moderate alcohol consumption -- their risks and benefits and the reactions to each of them -- offers a revealing glimpse into how American society's deep-seated, ambivalent and irrational attitudes toward alcohol may be killing hundreds of thousands of people each year.

Aspirin

The advice to "take an aspirin and call me in the morning" received new urgency in 1989 when a study of 22,000 physicians indicated that those who took one aspirin every other day had 44 percent fewer fatal heart attacks than doctors in the control group who took a placebo.

Today, cardiologists routinely advise patients at risk of heart attacks to take aspirin regularly. This advice is given despite the fact that aspirin -- the commonest drug in the United States -- can have serious side effects.

The doctors taking aspirin in the physicians study had* twice *as many sudden cardiac deaths,* twice *the incidence of moderate to severe hemorrhagic strokes and* almost twice *as many ulcers as those taking the placebo.

"Aspirin increases the risks of bleeding disorders, however, and can lead to gastrointestinal hemorrhage [bleeding] and even hemorrhagic stroke," said Dr. Curtis Ellison. "For individuals with a history of bleeding problems or ulcers, the risk of a hemorrhagic problem may exceed the potential benefits of taking aspirin to prevent a heart attack."

Dr. Dean Ornish, author of *Dr. Dean Ornish's Program For Reversing Heart Disease*, has even harsher words for aspirin. He points out that the doctors taking aspirin in the physicians study had **twice** as many sudden cardiac deaths, **twice** the incidence of moderate to severe hemorrhagic strokes and **almost twice** as many ulcers as those taking the placebo.

Dr. Ornish, who also serves as an assistant clinical professor of medicine and attending physician at the University of California, San Francisco Medical School, emphasizes that while "the group taking aspirin had fewer heart attacks, *overall* there was no difference between the two groups in number of deaths resulting from heart disease or from all causes of death."

Dr. Ornish's book is, on the whole, a very good and useful one; however his section on alcohol relies on a number of outdated studies which hamper the accuracy in this regard.

Despite powerful potential side effects (aspirin given to children or others with viral diseases can cause paralysis, brain damage or death), Americans rushed to their medicine cabinets and began swallowing aspirin at a prodigious rate.

Why? Because aspirin is a comfortable drug with which most Americans have grown up. It isn't associated with rowdy bars; aspirin abuse is not a visible societal problem which wrecks homes and causes accidents in which innocent people are likely to be injured or killed.

Aspirin isn't linked with evangelical Protestant and Muslim religious prohibitions against consumption.

In short, aspirin lacks the emotional baggage of alcohol.

The job for American society -- including government, industry and advocacy groups -- is to develop a rational policy that: (1) removes the negative emotional smears of alcohol to allow the majority of 90 percent to benefit from guilt-free moderate consumption while (2) protecting society and abuse-prone individuals from the harm of immoderation.

Alcohol May Save More Lives Than Aspirin

The emotional baggage attached to alcohol as a result of religious prohibition and abuse has made it almost impossible for the media and public policy makers to deal with it rationally. While 7 to 10 percent of Americans can't drink alcohol responsibly, public attitudes have been so thoroughly tainted that many of the remaining 90 percent of the population avoid even moderate drinking -- despite the fact that it could save many more lives than aspirin, with the added benefit that moderate drinkers may find such a lifestyle choice enjoyable.

As the numerous studies cited in this book point out, moderate alcohol consumers have a 40 to 50 percent lower risk of having or dying of a heart attack, a protective effect comparable to aspirin. However, moderate alcohol consumption goes aspirin one better since moderate drinkers have **at least a 10 percent lower death rate from all causes** than do abstainers.

But alcohol also has side effects: abuse is the most obvious and serious problem which must be enthusiastically attacked without depriving 90 percent of the population of alcohol's benefits.

And like aspirin, alcohol consumption has also been linked with increased incidence of strokes. However, numerous studies (such as the Boffetta and Garfinkel paper cited elsewhere) show that people drinking one or two drinks per day have **lower risk of strokes than abstainers.** Indeed, even drinkers who reported consuming more than

The stroke danger associated with alcohol lies in abuse, not use.

five drinks per day (in reality probably more due to under-reporting) showed a 40 percent greater risk than abstainers -- far less than the 200 percent increase for people taking one aspirin every other day. Yet anti-alcohol advocates continually rail about the stroke danger from alcohol while ignoring a common drug with five times the risk.

The stroke danger associated with alcohol lies in abuse, not use.

In comparing aspirin and alcohol, Dr. Ellison said, "An individual with a history of drug abuse, or even for a person who is ascertained to be at increased risk of alcoholism [such as a family history of abuse], the potential for harm from the use of alcoholic beverages may exceed the potential benefits."

The job for American society -- including government, industry and advocacy groups -- is to develop a rational policy that: (1) removes the negative emotional smears of alcohol to allow the majority of 90 percent to benefit from guilt-free moderate consumption while (2) protecting society and abuse-prone individuals from the harm of immoderation. The job so far has been a miserable failure.

Part II
Women, Alcohol & The Family

SEVENTEEN

Men, Women And Alcohol

Men and women are different.

This is not news; the quite prominent (add also valuable and often enjoyable) differences are apparent to most of us but not, it seems, to many medical researchers who continue to structure many of their studies around men.

Medical science seems to view research through glasses that make women mostly invisible. Regardless of the reasons, designing scientific research which includes more women has begun to increase only in the past five years or so.

Medical science seems to view research through glasses that make women mostly invisible.

In some very key areas pertaining to alcohol -- most notably coronary artery disease -- the cardio-protective effects of moderate drinking have been confirmed by studies on women. Moderate alcohol consumption works not only by increasing the "good" HDL cholesterol and decreasing the stickiness of blood platelets, but also by helping a woman's body convert some of her androgens (male hormones) into estradiol, the most prominent of the estrogen female hormones. This conversion of androgen offers a substantial degree of protection for heart attack risk in post-menopausal women.

In several other areas of great health significance to women, most notably in the areas of breast cancer and Fetal Alcohol Syndrome (FAS), **the science has been inconsistent, sensationalized in the media and frustratingly too incomplete for women to use in making personal health choices.**

Since a given "drink" will produce a higher blood alcohol concentration (BAC) in smaller people than larger ones, women's definition of "moderate" will, in general, be lower than a man's. These differences have important consequences for women.

The Important Differences

Women:

- ♥ produce more estrogens than androgens, which affect the course of many diseases, notably cardiovascular disease and many cancers;
- ♥ are, on average, 15 percent smaller than men;
- ♥ have a higher percentage of their body weight as fat: 25 percent as compared with 15 percent for men and
- ♥ have a smaller percentage of body fluids: 50 percent as opposed to 60 percent.

These differences have important consequences for a woman's drinking habits. Since a given "drink" will produce a higher blood alcohol concentration (BAC) in smaller people than larger ones, women's definition of "moderate" will, in general, be lower than a man's.

But body composition may also be an important concern. Since alcohol tends to concentrate in body fluids (and tends to avoid fat), the same drink may produce a higher BAC in a 145-pound woman than in a 145-pound man. However, individuals vary greatly in their ability to metabolize alcohol. As we mentioned earlier, women may also metabolize alcohol more slowly than men due to lower levels of alcohol dehydrogenase in their stomach linings.

As noted in this book's chapters on moderation and on cirrhosis, the peak concentration of blood alcohol **may** be the determining factor in alcohol's health effects with 0.046 BAC being some sort of threshold. This is only a hypothesis and needs more research to confirm or disprove.

Research also indicates that women:

- tend to absorb alcohol more rapidly at mid-cycle ovulation and just before menstruation;
- metabolize alcohol more slowly when they are taking birth control pills and
- who are alcoholics tend to develop more masculine characteristics due to atrophy of the ovaries.

Sperm counts can be decreased significantly at a level of abou four to five drinks per day on average which -- while producing normal sperm -- can affect overall fertility.

Reproductive Consequences For Men Too

Alcohol abuse by men also has consequences that have not been widely publicized. As the Porter commented to Macduff in Shakespeare's *Macbeth*, alcohol "provokes the desire but takes away the performance." This is, perhaps, the best known of alcohol's reproductive consequences and does not require a medical study to prove. It may also be nature's way of protecting future generations, because research has shown that high levels of alcohol can produce deformed sperm.

In addition, chronic male alcohol abusers:

- have higher estrogen levels;
- develop shrinking of the testes;
- lose pubic hair and develop feminine characteristics including enlarged breasts;
- are frequently impotent and
- lose the ability to produce sperm (deformed or otherwise).

Sperm counts can be decreased significantly at a level of about 50 grams of alcohol per day (about four to five drinks per day on average) which -- while producing normal sperm -- can affect overall fertility.

> ***"At best they [women] will suffer the anxiety that even moderate normal activity can damage their real or potential offspring. At worst, women will be treated as walking wombs, perpetually pregnant until proved otherwise, with pregnancy police peeping in at every door and restricting every activity -- except when they need them cheap."***— Stellman & Berlin

Why The Focus On Women?

Why have the media, the government, and the alliance among advocacy groups and religious organizations focused on women and not men? It could be just one more way to keep women barefoot and pregnant according to an article co-authored by Jeanne Mager Stellman, associate professor of clinical public health at Columbia University and Joan E. Berlin, associate director of the Women's Rights Project of the American Civil Liberties Union. In their article, first published in the June 4, 1990, *New York Times*, the writers said that the results of junk science and media sensationalism "can be awesome. At best they [women] will suffer the anxiety that even moderate normal activity can damage their real or potential offspring. At worst, women will be treated as walking wombs, perpetually pregnant until proved otherwise, with pregnancy police peeping in at every door and restricting every activity -- except when they need them cheap.

"Women's drinking and birth defects are big news," the women said, citing a *New York Times* Sunday magazine article which said that even a single drink during pregnancy could cause FAS and birth defects.

"But the research upon which these broad generalizations are based shows no such thing," Stellman and Berlin said. "In one set of studies, the authors [of the magazine article] clearly state that their data could not be interpreted below a three-drink-per- day level. They noted, moreover, that the 'strongest predictors of a child's IQ were other factors: 'maternal education, mother- infant interaction, paternal education, race and birth order.' Is it the occasional glass of wine or social factors...that should have been highlighted?"

Stellman and Berlin charged the media with ignoring men's reproductive issues. "The discussion of women and alcohol shows that bias still taints journalism and the interpretation of science. Today, we ridicule the notion that it was once 'scientifically' demonstrated that women are less intelligent because of smaller brain size and that education made women infertile. Pseudoscientific theories about poor blood, watery muscles and brain 'lateralization' have all been asserted to 'prove' women's biological and social weakness."

"Science does not grow from 'factlets' dripping from laboratory spigots; research is more than 'Eureka' in bathtubs -- no matter how many reporters record the event. Science is the accumulation of verifiable knowledge."

Unfortunately, as you will read in this book (and experience in our largely techno-illiterate media) the alcohol-control alliance is not beyond using "junk science" to advance its agenda.

"We've become a society drunk not on alcohol but on random 'factlets' wrested from scientific journals before the ink has dried," wrote Stellman and Berlin. "Science does not grow from 'factlets' dripping from laboratory spigots; research is more than 'Eureka' in bathtubs -- no matter how many reporters record the event. Science is the accumulation of verifiable knowledge."

In their article, the two women cite evidence that junk science is still being used against women.

"... even the prestigious *New England Journal of Medicine* recently [in 1990] ran a widely reported editorial emphasizing the relative inability of the female digestive system to metabolize alcohol efficiently compared with the male. These grandiose conclusions were based on a study of 20 men and 23 women -- 12 of whom were alcoholics and all of whom were hospitalized for gastric dysfunction!

"Where was the usual caution and prudence in the *New England Journal* over the over-extrapolation of data from hospitalized patients to the healthy population, and why was this story front- page news?

A Nevada woman lost custody of her newborn child because she drank some beer the day she went into labor. Since hospital workers smelled alcohol on her breath, she now has to prove herself a fit mother.

"The assertions about women's biology in general, and their role as child bearers, now threaten our civil liberties and the gains we have made."

The article cites two cases:

(1) A Nevada woman lost custody of her newborn child because she drank some beer the day she went into labor. Since hospital workers smelled alcohol on her breath, she now has to prove herself a fit mother.

(2) A pregnant Wyoming woman was jailed for prenatal child abuse when police smelled alcohol on her breath when she went to them seeking protection from an abusive partner.

In a more recent case in 1991, two waiters in a Seattle restaurant were fired after they harassed a pregnant woman who ordered a single mixed drink. The woman, who was then overdue for delivery, was subjected to a harangue about the hazard she was presenting to her unborn child; the waiters' diatribe included thrusting a government warning from a beer bottle in the woman's face.

This seemed too extreme even for Michael Jacobson, who heads one prominent alcohol-control advocacy group, The Center For Science In The Public Interest, which has helped to whip up much of the anti-alcohol hysteria. In an interview with *Wine Business Insider* shortly after the incident, Jacobson stressed that "she seems to have been a good girl" by abstaining during the rest of her pregnancy and that, in his opinion, she was entitled to this one alcoholic beverage since the baby had gone to full term.

There are a number of "good girls" who feel they ought not to require the permission of Jacobson, his organization, or any other "public interest" group before making their own decisions.

EIGHTEEN

Alcohol And Breast Cancer

While cancer frightens us all, breast cancer occupies a special place in the pantheon of human horrors because it attacks not only a woman's body, but also a part of her physiology that -- rightly or wrongly -- helps her define herself.

So women who consume alcohol should look with concern and interest at medical research that indicates that even moderate alcohol consumption may be associated with an increased risk of getting breast cancer. But it may not be.

Even the best scientific minds find breast cancer and alcohol research muddled, flawed, inconclusive and incapable of supporting a definitive public health decision.

Breast cancer is such an emotional subject that the news media (who typically have no scientific background with which to make informed decisions on, or evaluate the credibility of, medical research) tend to sensationalize research results and present a fragmented and out-of-context image of the science. In this respect, women are not well served by the American media. As a result, women need to make the extra effort to gather a complete set of information themselves, consult with their physicians and make the necessary informed decision that cannot be made when relying solely on media reports. The chapter in this book on evaluating research will give you more tips on this process.

Research Presents A Muddled Picture

Even the best scientific minds find breast cancer and alcohol research muddled, flawed, inconclusive and incapable of supporting a definitive public health decision. Unlike studies which can support clear-cut decisions (such as the ones on the cardio-protective effects of moderate drinking), research on the association between alcohol and breast cancer is inconsistent, shows different results from one study to another

The majority of the more recent studies fail to show a relationship between breast cancer risk and consumption of two or fewer drinks per day. However, the theme established by the earlier studies remains: no conclusive trend has been found.

and is, on the whole, not reproducible in a manner which points to a scientific conclusion.

This is indicated by a review of 23 major studies conducted by Dr. Keith Marton who found that 12 indicated some positive relationship between moderate alcohol consumption and breast cancer, nine indicated no increased risk and two were so flawed that the results could not be reliably interpreted. Dr. Marton has recently updated his review, adding more studies. The majority of the more recent studies fail to show a relationship between breast cancer risk and consumption of two or fewer drinks per day. However, the theme established by the earlier studies remains: no conclusive trend has been found.

Please note that in this context, "positive" does not mean "good" but indicates that a relationship exists; a negative relationship means that no relationship exists. This may be somewhat confusing and this clarification will be repeated to help decrease the confusion.

Some of the nine studies showing no increased risk which Dr. Marton reviewed actually indicated some slight **decreased** risk of breast cancer in moderate drinkers, but he felt that the decreases might not be statistically significant.

If, to be safe, you choose to ignore the nine studies showing no relationship and focus on the 12 that do, you find that the increased risk for women consuming moderately is about 50 percent.

If these are the correct results (and as you will read below, many scientists believe they are **not accurate**), this means that a woman's lifetime chance of dying from breast cancer may increase about 4 percent, from 8 to 12 percent. However, Dr. Marton said that even if you accept the worst-case studies as valid, a woman who drinks moderately must balance the 4 percent higher risk of getting breast cancer against the 20 to 30 percent lower risk of dying of heart disease -- a net positive effect of 6 to 14 percent.

If you accept the worst-case studies as valid, a woman who drinks moderately must balance the 4 percent higher risk of getting breast cancer against the 20 to 30 percent lower risk of dying of heart disease -- a net positive effect of 6 to 14 percent.

"Many of these studies," Dr. Marton said, "do not account for other factors (other than alcohol) that might affect the risk of cancer."

For example, one study conducted by the U.S. Centers for Disease Control and published in the Sept. 24, 1983, issue of *Lancet* found no increase or a slightly decreased risk of breast cancer for moderate women drinkers (Relative Risk -- as compared to abstainers -- of 1.0 for beer drinkers, 0.9 for spirits drinkers and 0.8 for wine drinkers). In examining why its results varied from earlier research that indicated an increased risk, CDC researchers found that one study used women with ovarian and endometrial cancers as a control group. "However, our data indicate a possible **protective** [emphasis added] effect of alcohol consumption on the risk of endometrial cancer. We are currently investigating the hypothesis that the increased breast cancer risk observed by [these studies] may be due to alcohol's protective effect on endometrial cancer rather than its causal effect on breast cancer."

In other words, the control group -- the group against which the drinkers were compared -- was not properly chosen and this biased the conclusions. Because epidemiological studies like these involve the mathematical manipulation of hundreds of thousands of pieces of data, the strategies used to collect and analyze the data can introduce hidden biases.

This was pointed out in a 1988 analysis of two reports from the *New England Journal of Medicine*, conducted by Nathan Mantel of the Mathematics, Statistics and Computer Science Department at American University and published in the book, *Preventive Medicine.* Mantel found that the two 1987 studies (one by Schatzkin *et al* and the second

The apparent increase in breast cancers associated with alcohol in some studies may be linked not to alcohol, but socio-economics.

by Willett *et al*) which indicated a positive association between alcohol and breast cancer "did not inquire into other cancers, morbidities, mortalities or total mortality" and did not correct for other physical and lifestyle characteristics, particularly obesity, that could affect the research conclusions.

"Thus the drinkers and the nondrinkers did not start in at even levels as they might have in an ideal study. And if they were not starting at even levels, they could well have been starting at uneven predilection levels for breast cancer." Mantel called the studies "defective" because the needed data was not collected and said that "it would be irresponsible to lead women to believe that moderate alcohol consumption is dangerous."

Mantel also took a shot at the news media, charging that "journalists seem bound to make...unqualified interpretations."

Similar biases can be found in other studies which show positive relationships (meaning that a relationship exists). But biases are not the only problems that plague research into alcohol and breast cancer. Indirect associations may also be to blame for the positive relationships.

This may be true with alcohol and breast cancer. In the same 1988 *Preventive Medicine* textbook which published Mantel's analysis, a team of Veterans Administration physicians lead by Dr. Randall E. Harris, M.D., Ph.D., of the American Health Foundation, said that the apparent increase in breast cancers associated with alcohol in some studies may be linked not to alcohol, but socio-economics.

Their logic goes as follows:

(1) Alcohol consumption increases linearly with education. Only 39 percent of women with less than nine years of education call themselves drinkers; that rises to about 70 percent for women with 16 years of education.

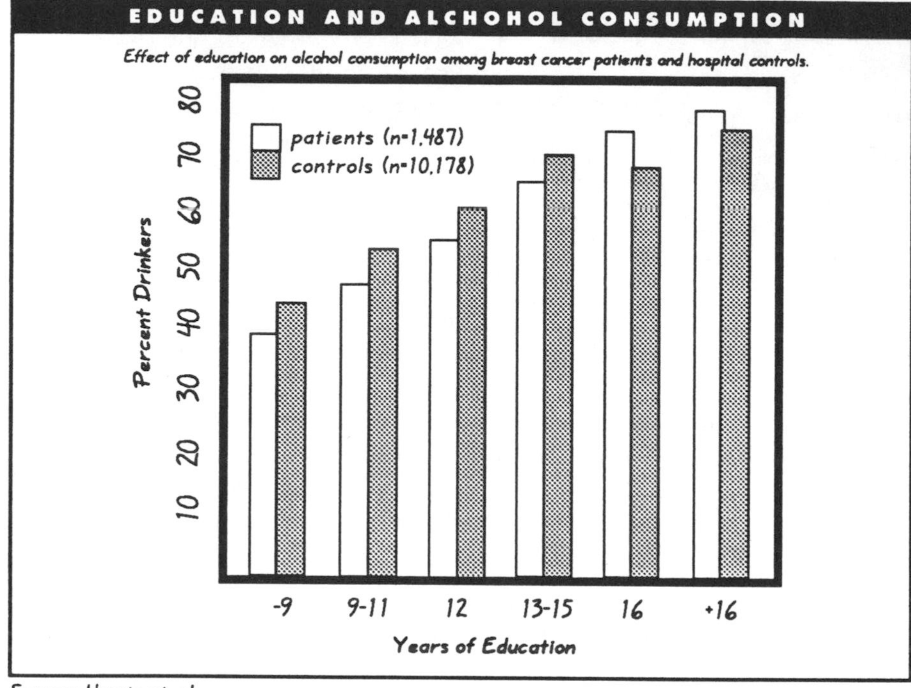

Source: Harris et. al.

(2) Well-educated women most often postpone pregnancies, often into their late 20s and 30s; less-educated women frequently have children in their teens.

(3) Breast cancer risk increases as the onset of the first pregnancy is postponed.

Therefore, the increased risk of breast cancer may be due to the postponement of pregnancy among educated women -- who tend to drink more and postpone pregnancy -- and not to alcohol consumption (which is perhaps only indirectly and not causally related).

Supporting this hypothesis is the fact that almost all of the studies which showed a positive relationship between alcohol and breast cancer showed the highest risk among thin drinkers. This is at odds with general data that shows obese women to be at higher risk for breast cancer. The explanation? Highly educated women (who drink more and who postpone their first pregnancy) tend to be

The increased risk of breast cancer may be due to the postponement of pregnancy among educated women—who tend to drink more and postpone pregnancy —(which increases breast cancer risk) and not to alcohol consumption itself.

thinner than less-educated women. Thinness, then, is also indirectly (but not causally) related to breast cancer.

However, thinness could be related in another way. The same amount of alcohol consumption would produce a higher level of blood alcohol in thin women than in those who are larger, thus accentuating the effects of alcohol.

Science simply has no conclusive answer on these hypotheses.

Because epidemiological studies such as these are subject to biases and indirect associations, one standard which scientists use to assess the credibility of the results is the presence of a logical biological mechanism. In other words, the most believable epidemiological studies are the ones which are backed up by laboratory studies (human or animal) which point to the **way** in which an agent like alcohol produces good or bad effects.

However, a biological mechanism to account for the possible breast cancer increases among moderate drinkers has **not** been discovered. In experiments on laboratory animals, there has been **no** association between alcohol and breast cancer.

Because of this lack of a plausible mechanism, the studies showing a positive association between breast cancer and moderate consumption are all suspect and may all be indirect associations.

Finally, the under-reporting of alcohol consumption which plagues epidemiological studies may mean that significantly larger amounts of alcohol (i.e., abuse) may be required to cause any increase in breast cancers.

How can a woman translate the studies into a personal decision relating to her own health? Decrease the chances of heart disease and increase (to a smaller extent) the risks of breast cancer or vice versa?

Women with a history of alcohol abuse or breast cancer in their families should be the most cautious since they are already at greater risk from these diseases.

The decision must be made not just on the scientific data, but on personal background and preferences. Women with a history of alcohol abuse or breast cancer in their families should be the most cautious since they are already at greater risk from these diseases. On the other hand, women without these factors may feel less constrained, especially if they particularly enjoy wine. Women who choose this option, however, should be aware that their smaller size means that the definition of moderate is set at a lower level than for men -- as is the level at which abuse begins.

What this means is that women must accept responsibility for gathering all of their information and making their own informed choices. They must also recognize that their needs are not served well by the news media which tends to sensationalize and make unqualified conclusions. Likewise, women should be skeptical of advocacy groups who may conceal information and distort research results in order to make statements about drinking behavior which support their positions.

NINETEEN

Wine, Pregnancy and Fetal Alcohol Syndrome

By Wells Shoemaker, M.D.

The distinctive features of both wine and women have lured ardent feminists, zealous prohibitionists, opportunistic politicians, and somber doctors to your dinner table ... without an invitation, and probably without a corkscrew.

Differences in physical size and metabolism have decreased the amounts of alcohol deemed "moderate" for women compared to men. Breast cancer and its potential relationship to alcohol, naturally, focus upon women, but nowhere is the gender emphasis so pointed as in the discussion of alcohol use during pregnancy.

It sounds simple to say that no pregnant woman **needs** to drink, and if there is any remote chance of harm, then "Just don't drink." The question remains just how "remote" are the risks, and what are the facts a woman should consider when making her personal decision.

The American fetus became a hot issue in the 1980s. The lawyers, the preachers, the politicians, the judges, and the doctors all wanted dibs on the unborn. At the same time, alcohol became a safe and popular target for this same cast of characters. The convergence of alcohol and the fetus produced a vortex of medical, legal and political interest in a relatively rare but poignantly tragic birth defect. Fetal Alcohol Syndrome (FAS) burst into national consciousness with a whirlwind exposure through every media channel.

PEDIATRICIAN'S NOTE

***"Jealously and forlornly, I wish we could direct similar energy and awareness* [such as that given to FAS] to basic pediatric preventive teachings, such as car seats, bike helmets, drownings, poisonings, burns and immunizations, which affect a hundred-fold more children."—WS**

The occurrence of FAS has been -- and continues to be -- overexaggerated and distorted by a number of anti-alcohol groups to stir up emotional support for their crusade.

Michael Dorris' moving book, *The Broken Cord*, received tremendous media attention as did a 1992 Congressional hearing chronicling the hardship of rearing an adopted Native American child with FAS.

Two Seattle restaurant employees earned national news notoriety in 1991 when their employer fired them for refusing to serve a drink to a pregnant woman several days past her delivery due date. This episode and the subsequent repercussions highlighted both the emotional intensity and the factual ignorance of the public's awareness about FAS.

As you read further, you'll see that the occurrence of FAS has been -- and continues to be -- overexaggerated and distorted by a number of anti-alcohol groups to stir up emotional support for their crusade. FAS is a serious, **preventable** tragedy which can be best eliminated through the use of solid facts, good science and sound public policy, rather than distortions and demagoguery.

What Is FAS?

FAS was first described in 1968 in France and then by a group of pediatricians in Seattle in the early 1970s, although it has probably existed since ancient times. In a clinic for learning disabled children, the Seattle doctors noticed a peculiar physical similarity among several of these children. They dug into the medical histories and then discovered that each child had an alcoholic mother.

Thousands of medical articles have been published on FAS since the original description, and the syndrome now consists of a constellation of features:

- Children with FAS are born small and never catch up;
- Their brains are small and underdeveloped;
- Their upper lips tend to be thin, and the *philtrum* (the ridges and groove that reach from the nostrils down to the upper lip) is often smooth or flattened;
- Their noses are short and upturned, and their eyes tend to be small, widely set, downturned, and sad looking;
- They resemble each other almost as if siblings and
- They have a statistical increase in other physical defects, particularly congenital heart disease.

***FAS children are generally exposed to ponderously abusive amounts of alcohol. We're not likely to be confused by "moderation" here. Typical ingestion histories range from two or three six-packs of beer or the better part of a fifth of distilled spirits* a day.**

The grittiest component of FAS is **mental retardation**, which tends to be severe and irremediable despite the best of modern educational interventions. The pathos of the wasted life of the innocent victim has earned FAS its deserved place among modern human tragedies, right along with babies who contracted AIDS from transfusions in hospital nurseries.

There is no X ray or laboratory test that establishes the diagnosis of FAS. Any of the separate physical or developmental components of FAS can be seen in other children, but when **all** or **most** of the features are present, along with a history of maternal alcohol abuse, an observant pediatrician can make the diagnosis.

How Much Alcohol Causes FAS?

FAS children are generally exposed to ponderously abusive amounts of alcohol. We're not likely to be confused by "moderation" here. Typical ingestion histories range from two or three six-packs of beer or the better part of a fifth of distilled spirits **a day**.

There have been no known cases of "full blown" FAS in children whose mothers consumed moderate amounts of alcohol; this is even

The typical profile of the FAS mother is a 30-plus-year old alcoholic in poor health, taking poor nutrition, smoking, living in a chaotic environment alone or in the company of a male alcoholic.

more telling considering that patients virtually always understate their alcohol intake. There have been no cases reported in which wine was the source of ethanol.

Clearly, there may be compounding factors that stress the fetus. The typical profile of the FAS mother is a 30-plus-year old alcoholic in poor health, taking poor nutrition, smoking, living in a chaotic environment alone or in the company of a male alcoholic.

Most of the organ systems in the human fetus develop in the first two months after conception, and it is likely that most of the physical malformations occur from early exposure to episodic, very high levels of alcohol (often from binge drinking or sustained high levels with daily intoxication, the latter being the most common pattern).

Physical growth of the fetus occurs throughout pregnancy, and the small size of FAS babies likely relates to toxic effects upon cell growth throughout the nine months. Brain growth accelerates markedly in the third trimester and cessation of maternal alcohol abuse before this point can considerably reduce the neurological handicaps of FAS.

Unanswered Questions

There remain some haunting medical questions to answer about FAS:

- A majority of heavily drinking mothers have babies with no identifiable abnormality.
- Some alcoholic mothers have delivered twins where one has FAS and the other seems normal.
- Some ethnic groups have a substantially higher incidence of FAS births; certain Native American groups have a 30-fold higher incidence than the general population.

It would be tremendously valuable, to guide both prevention and therapy, to determine what separates the fortunate from the afflicted.

The incidence itself is still controversial. While some professionals in the field claim that 1 or 2 babies per 1,000 births suffer FAS, data collated from 50 state health departments in the United States reveals the recorded occurrences are closer to 1 in 10,000. FAS researchers hasten to point out that the latter figure may be falsely low because American medical professionals overlook or misdiagnose 90 percent of all FAS cases. The truth probably lies somewhere between the two figures.

While some professionals in the field claim that 1 or 2 babies per 1,000 births suffer FAS, data collated from 50 state health departments in the United States reveals the recorded occurrences are closer to 1 in 10,000. FAS researchers hasten to point out that the latter figure may be falsely low because American medical professionals overlook or misdiagnose 90 percent of all FAS cases. The truth probably lies somewhere between the two figures.

The most carefully drawn studies suggest an intermediate figure of 1 in 3,000 births.

Experienced pediatricians traveling in Mediterranean countries have not noticed large numbers of FAS children, despite the fact that wine consumption may be tenfold higher than in the United States, and that pregnant women often continue drinking wine with their meals. National statistics do not reveal the elevated FAS occurrences that anti-alcohol activists would predict, and it's presumptuous to assert that Italian, French, Greek and Spanish doctors are less alert than American doctors.

In addition, statistics from those countries and the United States indicate that more alcohol is sold and consumed in the holidays that occur in the months of October through December. If these statistics are accurate, and if FAS is connected to alcohol consumption at **any** level, then we might expect to see increased incidences of FAS in births that occur from June to August. In fact, no such increase has been shown in any data.

This should offer consolation to women who have consumed alcohol at Thanksgiving, Christmas or Chanukah celebrations but who were unaware of their pregnancies.

Considerable research shows that the women who have taken FAS warnings to heart have been educated, middle-to-upper income women who were at substantially lower risk of FAS to begin with. There is no research at all which indicates that scare tactics have changed anything for women most at risk.

Fetal Alcohol "Effect"

Clearly and without controversy, abusive alcohol consumption during pregnancy is risky. Is it not plausible that some less extreme amount of consumption could cause fetal injury of a more subtle nature? It certainly seems logical that there should be some dose-effect between perfectly normal and overtly abnormal.

Fetal Alcohol Effect was coined to define a cluster of behavioral problems in alcohol-injured children who did not have the physical appearance of FAS. These include fidgetiness, short attention span, coordination problems, learning disabilities, and impaired social interactions.

PEDIATRICIAN'S NOTE

Newborn babies look wrinkled, red, squeezed, and gooey when they're born, (unless, of course, they're yours). Truthfully, subtle abnormalities of newborn facial features are hard to call. The wisdom of the modern health care system boots these babies and mothers out of the hospital in 24 hours, and a little flattening of the philtrum can certainly escape a very good doctor. Alcoholic mothers and their babies often drift from clinic to clinic for sporadic care, usually illnesses only. It's quite rare for one doctor to see them over a stretch of time. FAS often will not be suspected until preschool age. --WS

None of these traits are unique to alcohol-injured children and all can be found at some time in practically any child under stress.

In addition, some studies have tried to associate moderate alcohol consumption with lower birth weights or slightly lower IQ measurements; the overall body of scientific research shows **no** connection at all.

Some studies have tried to associate moderate alcohol consumption with lower birth weights or slightly lower IQ measurements; the overall body of scientific research shows no connection at all.

For example, Dr. Keith Marton surveyed 10 major research studies which looked at moderate alcohol consumption in pregnant women and birth weight. Of the 10 studies, six found no association at all; two found that children of mothers who drank moderately during pregnancy may have weighed slightly more than abstainers; two (which studied about 500 children, compared to the previous eight studies which examined about 62,000 children) found that abstainers had slightly smaller children. **Taken as a whole, these ten studies indicate that moderate consumption does not affect birth weight**.

The same situation exists in studies that looked at small variations in IQ. The vast body of research shows no association between IQ variations and moderate alcohol consumption by pregnant mothers; a small number say moderate drinkers' children may have IQs as much as five points higher than abstainers, while one other investigator, who has performed several studies, asserts just the opposite. Even these latter studies show no effect below three drinks per day **throughout** the pregnancy -- a level that most mothers would avoid simply because the taste of alcohol is unappealing.

In addition, psychologists generally agree that IQ measurement is imprecise and that five points is smaller than the margin of error on such tests. Finally, numerous examinations of IQ tests have proved that they are flawed by ethnic and economic biases which means that -- regardless of drinking patterns -- children of mothers who are at highest

PEDIATRICIAN'S NOTE

School problems can do more harm to a child's future than broken bones, ruptured appendices, and lobar pneumonia. No conscientious doctor can take learning and behavior problems lightly, even if the "testing instruments" are not perfect. —WS

risk (poor, Hispanic or African-American) will generally test lower on IQ tests than white, middle or upper-middle class women.

None of the FAE traits can be weighed or measured with a "hard" quantitative test, such as a blood test for diabetes or a urinalysis for a bladder infection. While experienced child psychologists can make helpful qualitative observations to guide the educational interventions for a troubled child, most behavioral tests incorporate a subjective component and considerable variation exists between different examiners.

Finally, many studies that have indicated a connection between FAS or FAE and moderate drinking have been seriously flawed in their methodology. In an article published in the September 1991 issue of the *British Journal of Addiction*, alcohol researcher Genevieve Knupfer showed that those studies that found a connection between moderate drinking and FAS were those which did not discriminate between moderate consumption and binging. For the purpose of these studies, a woman who drank 10 drinks at one sitting was identical to a woman who drank less than one drink per day over the course of a week.

"An examination of the research literature on the results of drinking during pregnancy does not provide any evidence that light drinking is harmful to the fetus," said Knupfer.

All of this means that professionals evaluating problem children face a troublesome temptation to overdiagnose FAE; if the question to them is phrased, "Is this problem consistent with FAE?", the entity is so amorphous that the answer will almost always be "Yes, possibly." Our society seems to want to fix the **blame** for most things and it is easier (if incorrect) to point at FAE than to try to alter structural problems in dysfunctional families -- problems whose magnitude totally overwhelms those of suspected FAE cases.

The bias to blame FAE looms larger when studies are designed to:

- be published for "ammunition" in the anti-alcohol campaign or
- justify continued funding from a granting agency which philosophically seeks to expand the public perception of alcohol- related injury.

The only way FAS is going to become truly preventable is to provide alcoholic mothers access to prenatal care, a scandalous impossibility for many in the United States. Meanwhile, anti-alcohol activists use FAS to scare the people who consume moderately and condemn the people who make alcoholic beverages.

Where to Draw the Line?

Fetal alcohol effect probably does exist, although once again at consumption levels any non-alcoholic person would instinctively shun. The crucial question for millions of mothers is, "What is the risk of an occasional drink? Is it true that even small consumption may damage my baby?" The answer usually comes shrink- wrapped with a legal or a political package, rather than a strictly medical one.

Reported in *Time* in August 1989, Dr. Robert Sokol, head of the federally-funded fetal alcohol research center at Wayne State University in Indiana, said, "Our best evidence is that we cannot detect adverse consequences to very light drinking, but that doesn't mean they don't exist."

Dr. Sokol's conservative stance is generally extrapolated by federal health and alcohol bureaus to a simple: "No drinking is safe." But is that true?

Through the 1980s all of the data for FAS and FAE had been gathered retrospectively, with an inherent bias in data collection caused by identifying affected children and then looking back to make connections. Since incidence claims vary widely, and since much of

Sorting Out The Studies

A prospective *study identifies a group of subjects in advance, characterizes and measures them, then evaluates the results after an interval of time. If they are subjected to an experimental intervention, the study is called a controlled trial. Results of prospective studies tend to be highly reliable, but they require considerable organization, manpower, and expense.*

Retrospective *studies look at events that have already occurred and try to make sense of why they happened. While useful as a first step, and sometimes opening the door to crucial new understanding,retrospective studies are notoriously vulnerable to errors because of bias in data collection, coincidences, and unrecognized influences. Tentative conclusions from retrospective studies generally must be subjected to a prospective analysis before they can be accepted as scientifically confirmed.*

A prospective study would take about 1,000 women of varying age and ethnicity, assign them randomly to different alcohol consumption programs, monitor them through pregnancy, and then follow the offspring through childhood and school. Ethically, of course, it would be impossible to do such a study in a Western democracy, much less fund it.

the data is not quantitative, it seemed several years ago that the only way to determine a true dose versus incidence risk would be to do a prospective study.

There appeared to be an impasse. The proponents of the Just Say No, Zero-Tolerance doctrine had a full nelson on their critics. "We say we are right. Lives are at stake. You can't prove we are wrong, and you can't even try, so it's morally imperative that you take our view." The Zero-Tolerance attitude, however, does not serve American women well. In response to public educational efforts, the number of women in the United States drinking during pregnancy dropped from 30 percent to 20 percent between 1985 and 1988, according to a survey by the Centers for Disease Control, but 20 percent is still a large number.

PEDIATRICIAN'S NOTE

Eighteen months is an adequate interval to determine physical growth, assess most of the important motor development milestones, and identify some key language and social skills. Learning disabilities and some more subtle social interactions cannot be reliably assayed until elementary school age.

The median number of drinks consumed by the drinking mothers was only four per month. Do we really have legitimate medical data to lay a lifetime guilt trip upon these women?

An answer came the *British Medical Journal* in July 1991. Scottish research physicians Forrest and Florey published the first **prospective** study of maternal alcohol dose versus fetal outcome.

In the British health system, in contrast to our fragmented approach, all pregnant mothers in a given locale funnel through the same prenatal supervision. Families are less mobile and less likely than Americans to disappear from follow-up. This 100 percent enrollment makes the British approach a powerful epidemiological tool, eliminating the selective enrollment of individuals whose socio-economic status and other habits might bias the frequency of observed abnormalities.

Bordering upon the heretical, the investigators found that children of light drinkers actually fared better than the children of abstainers in all categories of the Scottish tests.

Forrest and Florey obtained alcohol consumption histories from 846 consecutive women and repeatedly verified the information through the series of prenatal visits. They subsequently studied 592 of the children up to 18 months age.

Forrest and Florey found no increase in alcohol injury indicators on motor or mental development until consumption reached twelve drinks per week, correlating with a 1988 retrospective study published in the *British Medical Journal* that proposed ten drinks a week as a threshold level.

Bordering upon the heretical, the investigators found that children of light drinkers actually fared better than the children of abstainers in all categories of the Scottish tests.

Forrest and Florey concluded, "**Pregnant women probably need not abstain from alcohol altogether as no detectable adverse relation was found between the child's mental and physical development and the mother's weekly consumption at levels in excess of 100 grams absolute alcohol.** However, to allow for a margin of safety and taking into account the findings of an earlier phase of this study on the immediate effects on the newborn, it is recommended that pregnant women should drink no more than eight units of alcohol a week, the equivalent of about one drink a day."

What does a responsible society do with this information? One conclusion is abundantly clear: **There is no legitimate reason to frighten, rebuke or abort the mothers who consume lightly.**

A second conclusion is that society -- or government -- really shouldn't be acting on this information. Counseling and decisions about personal health practices ought to belong in the confidence of a physician's office, not the billboard.

Regrettably, since all too many American mothers can't afford personalized medical care, the government is going to play a role. Indeed, it does.

Preventable by Decree?

The warning labels on your wine bottles and restaurant walls are successes for the anti-alcohol forces, but they probably have not prevented one single FAS birth.

Wayne State University professor Dr. Ernest Abel, M.D., in his 1990 text *Fetal Alcohol Syndrome*, states, "Prevention of FAS should be a simple matter involving public education. Advising women that drinking during pregnancy can be harmful to the developing fetus would seem a straightforward and simple matter... However, despite national, state, and local public education campaigns, there is no indication that these efforts have reduced FAS."

The mothers at risk for FAS aren't paying attention, which comes as no surprise to physicians experienced with the behavior of alcoholism.

Well-intentioned activists, as well as a few opportunists, harp upon FAS as the third leading birth defect and the **only preventable one**, e.g. simply by abstinence. That's a smug and frustrating attitude when it floats down to a real-life doctor dealing with real people in the real world.

The only way FAS is going to become truly preventable is to provide alcoholic mothers access to prenatal care, a scandalous impossibility for many in the United States. FAS will continue as long as alcoholic women are isolated, impoverished, under-nourished and deprived of access to the health care system. We need to offer psychological support and supervised therapy for the disease of alcoholism. And subsequently, we must refrain from abandoning this recovering mother after her politically-appealing fetus becomes another welfare neonate. Alcohol abuse and FAS will continue until we, as a society, are willing to spend real resources on behalf of human beings with the disease of alcoholism, not just decals and innuendo.

Meanwhile, anti-alcohol activists use FAS to scare the people who consume moderately and condemn the people who make alcoholic beverages.

PEDIATRICIAN'S NOTE

Let me get personal. Be absolutely honest with your doctor both about how much you drink and your anxieties about drinking. You will need more than the advice "just to stop," obviously, or else you already would have done so. There are many truly wonderful people and organizations to help you, and it really does make a difference if you stop, no matter how far along you are in pregnancy.

Exaggerating and distorting the risks of alcohol as a matter of public policy hinders the preventive potential of public health. It also insults the intelligence of women who wish to draw their own conclusions, based on all the facts, rather than accept a politically and governmentally controlled position on the effects of alcohol consumption. Transforming the issue of light consumption during pregnancy from a health issue into a moral or legal one -- to the point of using the inflammatory term "child abuse" -- will drive away the small but desperate minority who truly need help.

This Pediatrician's Recommendations

- ♥ Ideally, mothers should not drink during pregnancy.
- ♥ Mothers who do choose to drink should take no more than one drink a day, gradually, concurrent with a meal. Wine or beer would be preferable to distilled spirits.
- ♥ Exposure to any reputed fetal toxin carries the highest risk in the first trimester of pregnancy. Most women with morning sickness aren't enticed by a glass of wine, anyway.
- ♥ If a mother has difficulty limiting herself to a drink a day, or if there are occasional days when she drinks three or more, both she and her fetus have a problem that needs professional help.

TWENTY

Breastfeeding And Alcohol

By Wells Shoemaker, M.D.

After nine months of puffy ankles, low back pain, heartburn, and dreary abstention, a mother can finally see her baby smile. She can also return to the civilized pleasures of wine with supper ... or can she?

Lactation counselors, helpful grandmothers, and board certified obstetricians have all traditionally endorsed the use of beer or wine with meals for nursing mothers.

While professionals have debated the risks of moderate alcohol consumption for the fetus, no one questioned the safety of occasional alcohol use by breastfeeding mothers ... until recently.

Two studies, both published in the *New England Journal of Medicine*, have attacked this once-safe harbor:

(1) Ruth Little, Sc.D., and coworkers reported in 1989 that breastfed infants whose mothers used alcohol performed equally in mental tests at one year of age, but lagged behind in motor development when compared to the babies of non-drinkers.

(2) Julie Mennela, Ph.D., from the Monel Chemical Senses Center in Philadelphia, reported in 1991 that the milk of alcohol- consuming mothers had a different odor and was less appealing to infants.

As a pediatrician and founder of a hospital-based lactation program, I find serious flaws in both studies.

The Little group did not quantify nor verify the reported alcohol consumption among their mothers, nor did they define different types of beverages, the timing of drinking with meals, nor time of day.

They used standard developmental tests, but acknowledge that the tests "are not precise measures." Indeed, the scoring system does not measure a quantitative feature, such as weight or blood pressure. These scores are helpful to guide decisions for an individual, but are not legitimately designed to be added, divided, squared, and averaged by a statistician.

There are no population studies that remotely suggest any difference in growth of babies based upon mothers' alcohol consumption habits while nursing.

Accepting these limitations, what were the differences? The alcohol-exposed babies scored 98 and the others 103 on a motor test. This corresponds to approximately a one week difference in the age at walking, when the norm extends from 9 to 15 months.

As the author states in her conclusion, "What is the clinical importance of these findings? For the individual child, probably none."

The Monel Chemical group, which has also published their data on garlic odors in breast milk, studied a dozen women and reported their odor assessments after mothers drank a measured amount of alcohol.

The *New England Journal* subsequently published a sound repudiation of this study in the correspondence section, stressing the biological implausibility of the minute amounts of alcohol having any effect and the lack of any objective measurement of aromatic differences, even with highly sensitive instrumentation. Furthermore, there are no population studies that remotely suggest any difference in growth of babies based upon mothers' alcohol consumption habits while nursing.

Let's Calculate

Let's do some arithmetic, deliberately skewed to maximize the amounts of alcohol that could reach a breastfeeding baby.

Let's say a mother drinks to the point of intoxication with a blood alcohol content (BAC) of 0.10. Let's say the alcohol passes from the blood into the mother's milk immediately and with equal concentration (both assumptions are exaggerations). The mother's milk will have 0.1 grams of alcohol in 100 ml (about 3 1/2) ounces of milk.

Let's say her typical 11 pound (5 kg) two month old baby drinks a typical 4-ounce quantity of breast milk. Let's assume that the baby absorbs the alcohol from the milk immediately and completely into the bloodstream (a considerable exaggeration). The baby will have a BAC of about 0.002 -- too low to have any recognized pharmacological effect.

The real threat is that babies raised by intoxicated mothers face serious risks of being injured, burned, abused, malnourished and neglected.

Now let's eliminate the physiological exaggerations. Let's have the mother drink one glass of wine or beer, rather than three or four. Let's have her take this with a meal, which will both delay the absorption and reduce the level of alcohol in her blood and her milk. In this more realistic case, the baby will achieve a BAC well below 0.001 -- too low to measure with conventional instruments.

The Pediatrician's Recommendation

Two of nature's most eloquent triumphs in the liquid phase are mother's milk and fine wine. Mothers should provide the former in abundance and consume the latter in moderation.

There are no realistic scientific reasons to discourage truly moderate, healthy, nursing mothers from occasional beer or wine with meals, but there certainly is a dark side of alcohol and motherhood.

Abusive consumption of alcohol might conceivably cause some pharmacological effect on a baby, but that's still a minor issue. The real threat is that babies raised by intoxicated mothers face serious risks of being injured, burned, abused, malnourished and neglected.

The enemy is the disease of alcoholism. All citizens, winemakers and anti-alcohol crusaders alike, need to unite in the pursuit of meaningful solutions to this problem. Frightening or misinforming healthy mothers really will not save any souls, make babies walk earlier or smell better.

TWENTY-ONE

Keeping Youth From Abusing Alcohol

Teenagers drinking alcohol isn't much of a problem in Italy or France or in other Mediterranean countries. Oh, they **do** drink; it's just not a major problem like it is in the United States.

The U.S. has a problem with teenage drunk-driving slaughter, many experts believe, because Americans seem unable to teach moderation and responsible use to their children. Like so many things, most Americans see drinking as all-or-nothing, good- versus-bad, black-or-white, yes-or-no and no "maybe" allowed.

U.S. government policy and most cultural mores urge a "Just Say No" attitude to both sex and alcohol. As a result, American kids are naive and ignorant about sex and alcohol -- which together often produce their own spontaneous combustion. It should come as no surprise that the United States has the highest teen pregnancy rate in the Western world along with the highest teen AIDS population as well as more teenagers who are killed and maimed by alcohol abuse.

Teaching youth about drinking alcohol is a lot like teaching them about sex. In America many people feel that teaching kids about sex is the same as teaching them to have sex; that showing them which end of a condom to use is the same as urging them to use it. U.S. government policy and most cultural mores urge a "Just Say No" attitude to both sex and alcohol. As a result, American kids are naive and ignorant about sex and alcohol -- which together often produce their own spontaneous combustion. It should come as no surprise that the United States has the highest teen pregnancy rate in the Western world along with the highest teen AIDS population as well as more teenagers who are killed and maimed by alcohol.

Does Ignorance Have to Continue to Kill Teenagers?

Most French and Mediterranean youngsters grow up with wine on the dinner table and are introduced to small amounts of it (diluted with water) frequently by the age of 10. As Dr. Wells Shoemaker puts it, he found that in that part of the world, wine is "a matter-of-fact, pleasant, unpretentious part of the evening meal. It wasn't a 'score' that I had to make with a fake ID in a liquor store. It wasn't a sexual thrill, and it wasn't a macho overture. It was supper."

> ***In the Mediterranean, wine is "a matter-of-fact, pleasant, unpretentious part of the evening meal. It wasn't a 'score' that I had to make with a fake ID in a liquor store. It wasn't a sexual thrill, and it wasn't a macho overture. It was supper."***—Wells Shoemaker

There is much support for the premise that parents who teach their children about alcohol **in the home**, and teach them pragmatically about moderation and responsibility, will dramatically decrease the risk of abuse outside the home -- along with the sometimes tragic consequences that result.

"Many who have studied the etiology [course of development] of alcoholism, believe that the complete prohibition of exposure to alcoholic beverages until 'adulthood' is not an appropriate way of preventing alcohol abuse," wrote Dr. Curtis Ellison, M.D., in his editorial in the September 1990 issue of the medical journal, *Epidemiology.*

"We expect to raise these people [children] to the age of 21, open the door and say, 'Now drink; it will be fine dear.' And of course, we know how badly that has failed," said Dr. Margaret Deansley, M.D., a practicing physician affiliated with the Stanford Medical School and a widely known lecturer on both alcohol abuse and breast cancer. "So, I am very much an advocate of making it [education in responsible drinking] an acceptable part of the home curriculum, and if necessary, the school's, " she continued.

But because the official U.S. government alcohol policy is abstinence, voices like those of Drs. Deansley, Ellison and Shoemaker and even research studies which do not concur with the official position find no recognition within the agencies.

One such report was a 1986 study, *The Minimum Legal Drinking Age and Traffic Fatalities*, funded by the National Institute on Alcohol Abuse and Alcoholism (NIAAA). That report concluded, "Our findings with respect to the minimum legal drinking age and drinking experience are not happy ones for public officials. It does not appear that the high fatality risk presented by new drinkers can be ameliorated by raising the legal drinking age.... The problem arises not because we permit people to drink when they are 'too young,' but rather because we permit them to experience the novelty of 'new drinking' at a time when they are legally able to drive. If drinking experience preceded legal driving, a potentially important lifesaving gain might follow."

The problem arises not because we permit people to drink when they are 'too young,' but rather because we permit them to experience the novelty of 'new drinking' at a time when they are legally able to drive. If drinking experience preceded legal driving, a potentially important lifesaving gain might follow.

The authors were correct that their findings were not happy ones for public officials; theirs, and other studies which have reached similar conclusions, conflict with official policy and have been both ignored and suppressed by NIAAA and its parent agency, the Department of Health and Human Services (HHS). Researchers, who are funded by such very politicized agencies as NIAAA, and even some units of the National Institutes of Health, learn very quickly that their study grants dry up when they produce conclusions that conflict with official policy.

But not every agency in the federal government has ignored studies that run counter to the "no-use, just-say-no" policy on alcohol. This policy was blasted in 1991 by the General Accounting Office (GAO) which serves as an investigation arm of Congress. The GAO issued a report critical of the HHS, the Department of Education and HHS's Office for Substance Abuse and Prevention (OSAP).

The GAO study said that the no-use policy of those agencies does not work and further that their deliberate linking of alcohol with illegal drugs in order to make alcohol look bad was "unacceptable" and perhaps counterproductive and detrimental.

Instead, the GAO report urged more emphasis on responsible decision-making approaches in order to decrease risky behavior, not only for teenagers but for all Americans.

The GAO study said that the no-use policy of those agencies does not work and further that their deliberate linking of alcohol with illegal drugs in order to make alcohol look bad was "unacceptable" and perhaps counterproductive and detrimental. Instead, the GAO report urged more emphasis on responsible decision-making approaches in order to decrease risky behavior, not only for teenagers but for all Americans.

How Bad Is The Problem?

Government agencies and private advocacy groups regularly issue news releases and hold seminars on how the teen drinking problem is getting worse and worse and why they need ever-increasing funding to fight the growing menace.

But government statistics themselves show that the situation is getting better, not worse. Some examples:

- ♥ A survey conducted by the National Institute on Drug Abuse (NIDA) shows that from 1979 to 1990, the proportion of 12- to 17-year-olds who ever drank alcohol declined by 31 percent and that from 1982 to 1990, the proportion of 18- to 25-year-olds who reported ever having consumed alcohol dropped by 17.4 percent.

- Binge drinking (defined as five or more drinks at a single drinking session) declined 21.8 percent from 1980 to 1990 according to a study conducted by NIDA along with the University of Michigan's Institute for Social Research.

Government statistics show that the situation of youth alcohol abuse is getting better, not worse. Binge drinking (defined as five or more drinks at a single drinking session) declined 21.8 percent from 1980 to 1990 according to a study conducted by NIDA.

This is not to say, in any way, that abuse among American youth can be ignored. It does say that government agencies and advocacy groups, whose financial funding and jobs depend on the continuation of a serious problem, will sometimes distort the truth.

The job then falls to parents to level with their children, tell them the truth about alcohol's dangers and its potential for the social and health benefits which can come from **responsible, moderate consumption.**

How Do You Teach Responsibility?

Dr. Deansley said that her approach to teaching her children about alcohol was much the same as she used in teaching them how to decrease other risky behaviors.

In her own words: *"I raised my children in the typical fashion, and that is to say that when they were in diapers, they were in the backyard with me. When they could understand me and could be with me by the hand, they could be in the front yard and when they were older, they were allowed to go as far as the front gate but not out into the street.*

"When they started going to school, there were very careful arrangements for their passing down the street and there was a crossing guard to help them to the safety of the school yard to protect them from traffic. As they grew older, they went to driver's training and they drove with a parent for a measured period of time prescribed by law and they took a test prior to doing that and then I kept my eye on the odometer and knew whether the car which we had allowed them to use, had in fact just gone down the street to meet friends for a hamburger or in fact

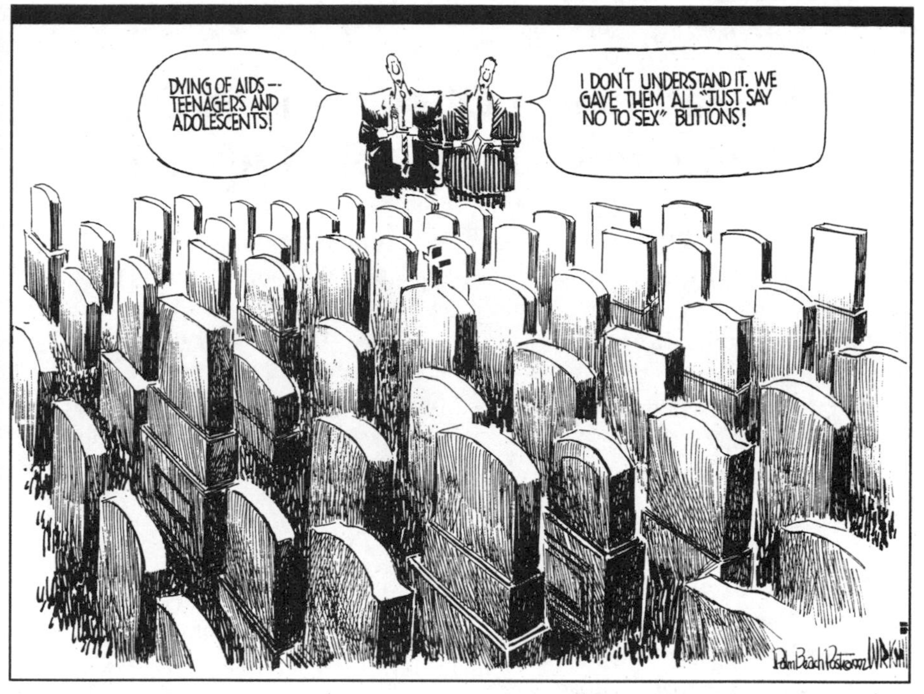
DYING OF AIDS -- TEENAGERS AND ADOLESCENTS!
I DON'T UNDERSTAND IT. WE GAVE THEM ALL "JUST SAY NO TO SEX" BUTTONS!

had disappeared twenty miles and had come back in rather record time because it had to be accomplished during the time allotted for a hamburger.

"What I am saying is that I taught my children about behaviors which might have risks in a graded fashion. These are typical teaching patterns of families against potential risk behaviors. Unfortunately, these are not patterns which are advocated, offered, sanctioned or are socially acceptable when it comes to alcohol consumption in our society, presently."

Deansley said parents need to teach their children about alcohol in the same graduated way that they ought to with other behaviors which involve a degree of risk.

Sidebar Eleven

A Pediatrician's Observations On Preventing Youth Alcohol Abuse

By Wells Shoemaker, M.D.

Children who develop a balanced view of drinking, by observing responsible models and trying alcoholic beverages in a safe and traditional mealtime setting, will be less likely to endanger themselves and others by impetuous consumption as young adults.

There is no creature on the planet more resourceful than an American high school senior who has been told there is something he cannot do. We glorify this trait in young-hero movies, but we may also confront a dangerous face of this same character on the way home from the movie theater.

Teenagers can and will obtain prohibited materials and engage in prohibited activities as long as they represent:

- ♥ a challenge to their creative energies, especially where their success can be recognized by peers,
- ♥ access to pleasures and thrills defined as "adults only" and
- ♥ symbolic demonstration of independence from parents and authority.

Teenagers who obtain alcoholic beverages commit what our society considers a criminal act. The spoils need to be consumed surreptitiously, usually in some dumb place. They can't bring partial containers back, so they have to finish off the whole six-pack or the whole bottle. An automobile trip usually separates the drinking site from the safety of bed.

Teenagers learn a great deal from their parents in 15 years, although they may not be willing to say "Thank you." The consistent behavior of the adults close to a young person is the most influential of all educational devices, as actions speak more clearly than didactic words.

If parents use beverages in moderation, I suggest occasionally offering small portions of wine or beer to children in a mealtime setting. The young people will know what they taste like and discover that the drinks are not magic keys to super powers or mystical vision or sexual conquest. Coupled with the consistent demonstration of moderate behavior, this matter-of-fact approach strips away the adventurism which can lead impressionable young people to drink foolishly away from the safety of home and the grounding influence of the home environment.

Alcohol in School?

Alcohol deserves a place in the educational system. No, not in a glass, and not to encourage its use, but to understand its double-edged nature. Dogmatic condemnations of its use may stick for a little while, just as the McCarthy-esque "education" I received about Communism in the 1950s did. The trouble is that little kids grow up and begin to recognize lies, distortions, and hypocrisy. Betrayed, they often spitefully adopt diametrically opposed beliefs and behavior -- as our country witnessed in the late 1960s.

Many anti-alcohol groups consider that to present any face of alcohol other than the grievous vector of abuse will tacitly encourage youth to act abusively. This factually unfounded posture insults the intelligence of young people. Worse, it probably stimulates exactly what we all wish to avoid by giving alcohol an undeserved mystique as the "forbidden fruit."

What would constitute a realistic curriculum to form a base of information upon which young people could make responsible decisions?

- ♥ History of alcohol and its role in civilizations of the past: agricultural, economic, social, political, religious issues, including manifestations of abuse.
- ♥ Contemporary use of alcohol, comparative world cultural and religious approaches, from Islam to Ireland, Chablis to Chicago, Moscow to Miami, Tel Aviv to Timbuktu.
- ♥ Medical physiology of alcohol effects upon the healthy person as well as the health consequences upon abusers. Fetal alcohol syndrome. The medical "play by play" of a drunken evening, analyzed by organ systems.

- The sociological consequences of alcohol abuse upon the individual, the family, and society at large. Short term dangers, long term outcomes. The disease of alcoholism will affect 10 percent of these students at some point in their lives, often manifesting early in the teen years.

Teenage Alcoholics

Parents who use alcoholic beverages abusively may have given their children both the genetic predisposition and the behavioral model to follow their path. This situation may apply to 5 to 10 percent of American households. Children of alcoholics face exaggerated risks of dangerous behavior, both for themselves and for others, as well as a likelihood of unhappiness in life.

Teenage alcoholics are, in my opinion, some of the most scandalously under-served sick persons in our society. Many pediatricians are learning through their continuing education to recognize these individuals; however, pediatricians rarely have a chance to help. Educational exposure through the schools stands a chance to bring these young people closer to understanding and help before some awful trauma has occurred.

To Think About

"According to a special report by the National Department of Justice, of those people arrested for driving under the influence of alcohol only about "2 percent reported drinking only wine. . . " National Department of Justice, Bureau of Justice Statistics, "Special Report", 1988, p. 1.

Part III
The Science of Wine and Health

TWENTY-ONE

Avoiding Junk Science: How To Make Your Own Decisions About Scientific Studies

We live in an age of "junk" science where almost any industry or advocacy group can issue a "scientific" report they claim supports their own particular agenda. No matter how biased or frail the "study" may be, it can find a constituency among Congressional or state legislative committees, the media, or before cheering/screaming crowds who are true believers in whatever point the study claims to "prove."

This chapter will enable you to make your own decisions about the validity of "research" as presented in the media or by advocacy groups. You don't have to be a scientist to make good decisions, but you need to know what makes a valid study and what does not.

Why Is Public "Science" So Bad?

Junk science goes unchallenged, for the most part, because our increasingly technological society grows increasingly illiterate in science and technology. When citizens, public policy makers and members of the media are incapable of understanding and intelligently dealing with science, they all become easy pickings for junk science and technological demagoguery. The result is that important public policy decisions concerning science are frequently made based on emotions rather than fact.

Junk science goes unchallenged, for the most part, because our increasingly technological society grows increasingly illiterate in science and technology. When citizens, public policy makers and members of the media are incapable of understanding and intelligently dealing with science, they all become easy pickings for junk science and technological demagoguery.

Unfortunately, there are all too many ideologues ready to announce yet another "scientific" study that is, in reality, a thin veneer of credible-looking, pseudo-science wrapped around propaganda and hidden agendas.

Two classic examples of this are: (1) the tobacco industry's pack of nonsense and outright lies, presented to Americans for decades, insisting that tobacco didn't kill and (2) the environmental movement's over-reactive hype about Alar which turned out to be a non-danger, but nevertheless crippled apple farmers and discouraged Americans from eating one of nature's healthiest foods.

We all should be skeptical in viewing claims from either industry or advocacy groups. Both have a vested interest in distorting data, scientific or otherwise, to support their own agendas.

The media usually lacks the expertise to examine the scientific credibility of a study even if it had the time to devote to the task. So the result is that debates on public policy boil down to a "he said, she said" argument between two "scientific" positions that, to the scientifically unlearned, look mostly equal.

In these cases, the advocate group espousing the latest ideology -- that can stage a dramatic scene for television cameras in front of dying babies or other filmable scenes -- will win the battle. While it may make good theater, it makes for junk science and bad public policy making.

Good science can not be decided by public opinion polls or debate. Democracy is the best political system in the world, but a majority vote to repeal the law of gravity has no effect on the way that physics or biology or any other science really works.

Good science can not be decided by public opinion polls or debate. Democracy is the best political system in the world, but a majority vote to repeal the law of gravity has no effect on the way that physics or biology or any other science really works.

Junk science wins so frequently because good science rarely offers the unequivocal results that make good dogma. And the quiet, reasoned, cautious voices of good scientists frequently drown beneath the shouts of the true believer's zeal.

This has been true of alcohol issues since Prohibitionists vandalized and destroyed taverns with axes to the present day when the anti-alcohol lobby often distorts facts to support their ideological position.

Research" which is presented in dogmatic, unqualified, absolute, unequivocal terms should be viewed with suspicion because it is probably concealing the qualifiers in order to support a hidden agenda.

Making Informed Decisions

Health research is fraught with ethical dilemmas, the most important of which is when, how and if to experiment with human beings. Specific areas, such as new drug and medical treatment trials, have strict regulations and the results can be accurately judged.

But the study of lifestyle factors and how they relate to the health of millions of people is not so precise. This is especially true with chronic diseases like atherosclerosis and cancer. Because those diseases take so long to develop and not every person at risk contracts them, they are much more difficult to study. It is simply impractical -- not to mention unethical -- to put thousands of people in a laboratory in order to study their behavior and the resulting health outcomes.

The science of epidemiology studies these relationships. It tries to assess the "Relative Risks" of an individual developing a disease if he/she engages in certain conduct or possesses certain physical attributes.

Epidemiology is an *observational* science rather than an *experimental*. Ethics demand that, in most cases, scientists observe people and make conclusions based on those observations rather than perform experiments on them.

Epidemiology studies large populations (typically thousands or perhaps hundreds of thousands) and tries to draw "statistically valid" associations between the disease and certain risk factors.

It is simply impractical—not to mention unethical—to put thousands of people in a laboratory in order to study their behavior and the resulting health outcomes.

Thus a relative risk of 1 means the event is certain (the relative risk of death, for example) and a relative risk of 0 means the event cannot happen (living forever, for example). The closer the relative risk gets to 1, the more likely it is to happen.

But because epidemiology is a study of populations, it cannot -- with certainty -- predict that reducing relative risks will benefit a **specific** individual. Fastening your seat belt means you have decreased your relative risk of being injured in an automobile accident; it doesn't mean that **you** cannot be injured.

Epidemiology is less exact because many of its observations come from questioning people whose recall may be biased or incomplete. In addition, people who refuse to participate in the study may have some characteristic in common which biases the sample of participants and makes it unrepresentative of the population as a whole. Factors unaccounted for, including random statistical glitches, may bias the results.

How To Unmask Junk Science

As imperfect as epidemiology can be, techniques have been developed which increase accuracy and decrease bias. In addition, science has developed a number of "reality checks" that can be used to determine if studies -- epidemiological or otherwise -- are reliable.

You can unmask junk science yourself and determine the reliability of a scientific study by asking a few non-scientific questions.

Where was the research conducted?

Look for the name of a respected medical institution or university. Make sure the research was conducted **at** the institution rather than by someone who is (or was formerly) associated with it. Be cautious of "institutes" with unfamiliar but civic-minded names. Industry and advocacy groups have created hundreds of them to give junk science studies credibility and to hide particular agendas.

What are the credentials of the people who conducted the research?

In medical research, look for M.D. or a Ph.D. in the relevant scientific discipline. Junk science medical studies often lack M.D.s. They often have an unusually large number of Ph.D.s who have studied subjects peripherally related or totally unrelated to the science required by the study. A Ph.D. in sociology is rarely qualified to author an article on biochemistry.

In medical research, look for M.D. or a Ph.D. in the relevant scientific discipline. Junk science medical studies often lack M.D.s and often have an unusually large number of Ph.D.s in sociology or other non-hard-science areas. A Ph.D. in sociology is rarely qualified to author an article on biochemistry.

Were the results published in a respected medical or scientific journal?

Again, like "institutes", industry and advocacy groups have founded dubious "journals" to lend respectability to their junk science.

On the other hand, articles in journals like *Lancet, Journal of the American Medical Association, Science, Nature, Cardiology* and so forth have been extensively reviewed by panels of qualified scientists who examine them for accuracy and credibility. Beware that many of the advocacy journals have been similarly named with the intent to deliberately mislead.

How many people were in the study?

The more people in a study, the more likely that the study will be statistically valid. Beware of studies with only a few dozen people. The results are more likely to be biased or to produce spurious or indirectly associated results.

Was the study population properly selected?

A study on white males may, or may not, be valid for white or African American women. Beware of some hidden bias at work.

Is the relationship a spurious association?

A spurious association is one which seems to be valid, but in fact, is unrelated. Sometimes these result from random fluctuations in the data used and can produce false results. These can happen to the best scientists with the best intentions. This is one good reason you should not make a decision based on one study. Spurious associations are not repeatable by other teams at other times.

Is the association indirect?

In nineteenth century England, researchers found that cholera struck mostly in low- lying areas. They concluded the disease was carried by smelly contaminated air found in such places. But despite the impressive association that people living in low-lying areas got cholera (as compared to people living on mountain sides) scientists later discovered the disease was caused by bacteria in contaminated water.

Is there a plausible process to explain the study results?

Indirect and spurious associations can be eliminated by determining if the associations have a logical mechanism for action.

The search for a biological mechanism between sugar and heart disease turned up another indirect association back in the mid- 1960s. An early study turned up a link between sugar consumption and heart disease. But, as scientists looked for how sugar consumption affected the heart, they learned that cigarette smokers consumed far more sugar than non-smokers. It turned out that smoking was the real cause behind the increased heart disease and sugar was not the culprit, but was only indirectly linked.

Similarly, critics of some of the studies of the beneficial effects of moderate drinking have often charged that the beneficial effects must be due to something else. But the discovery that moderate consumption can increase "good" HDL cholesterol, and that increased HDL levels are related to lower heart attack risk, helps remove the effect from the indirect association category. Likewise, the discovery that moderate alcohol (like aspirin) decreases the tendency of blood to clot in the arteries offers another credible mechanism.

Valid decisions can be made only on data that has been confirmed in a wide variety of studies involving different populations, researchers and analytical methods. A valid decision cannot be made on the basis of a single study. It must be made by looking at the **overall** *body of research.*

Are the results consistent with the overall body of research?

Valid decisions can be made only on data that has been confirmed in a wide variety of studies involving different populations, researchers and analytical methods. As this book has stated numerous times, a valid decision cannot be made on the basis of a single study. It must be made by looking at the **overall** body of research.

For example, not every study of alcohol and health has shown the cardio-protective effects of moderate consumption. In 1989, Dr. Keith Marton reviewed 22 scientific papers that evaluated the associations between alcohol and deaths from coronary artery disease. Of the 22 papers, 16 demonstrated the lowest mortality in moderate drinkers, five showed no difference and one of them focused on heavy drinkers only and was not relevant to moderate drinking. A closer examination of the five studies showing no difference indicated flaws that biased the studies toward their conclusions.

Since 1989, **every** major study (such as those by Klatsky at Kaiser Permanente Medical Center in Oakland, Calif., and by Rimm at the

Harvard University School of Public Health) have demonstrated significantly lower death rates among moderate drinkers.

Is the effect dose-related?

If more of a given factor produces more (or less) of a disease, the factor is said to be dose-related. Such a dose-related relationship is further evidence that the factor being studied is the **cause**.

In the case of alcohol and most pharmacueticals including antibiotics and aspirin, the dose relationships can be charted by J-shaped curves. In these cases none or little of the substance causes little or no effect; increasing the dosage increases the benefits. But at some point, the benefits begin to decrease and side effects appear. With most antibiotics and pharmacueticals, some vitamins and with alcohol, too much of a good thing becomes toxic.

Dose relationships give the lie to many advocacy positions which say that if high levels of a substance are proven harmful, then even extremely low levels of the substance are also harmful. For example, anti-alcohol groups say that since drinking five bottles of wine a day is unhealthy (no argument!) then drinking a quarter of a bottle a day is also unhealthy. This is simply untrue and scientifically invalid. In **some** cases, with **some** substances, it **may** be possible to extrapolate results like this, but not always and not with alcohol.

Is The Study Based on Original Data or Research?

Junk science can often be disguised in papers filled with footnotes which seem to be valid articles. However, a closer examination often reveals that the article's conclusions are based on old, outdated or unreliable data sometimes taken out of context. At other times, the data is taken third-hand from other government agencies without regard for the accuracy with which it was collected.

Finally, one of the most common ways of making junk science appear to be valid is for a small group of people working in the same field to "swap attribution." In other words, if I write an article which is supported by a shred of data and a seat-of-the-pants opinion, and a friend quotes the article or uses it as a footnote, it gives my article legitimacy while making his article seem like it is quoting a valid scientific study. Next, I can write another article which cites this last one by my friend (and perhaps a few other friends who are doing the same thing). My friends and I write a lot of articles like this which means we get to list a lot of footnotes which give the illusion that any given article is based on a great deal of research.

When making decisions affecting your health, place your trust in M.D. doctors, not in the Ph.D. "doctors" who are so frequently better versed in social engineering and politics than in medicine.

Alcohol abuse pioneer and Yale professor Selden Bacon has accused people in the anti-alcohol movement of doing just this sort of attribution swapping to lend an air of scientific legitimacy to poorly conducted research which may be without basis at all. Many "journals" in the alcoholism field are filled with articles of this sort.

This is a far cry from respectable, credible scientific publications like the *Journal of The American Medical Association* and its companions which require rigorous research, original data -- all of which are peer-reveiwed by medical and scientific experts.

Sidebar Twelve

"Proving" a Scientific Impossibility

The anti-alcohol movement didn't invent junk science, but instead follows in some very well-trodden footsteps. Some of the most fertile ground for junk science is the *indirect association* -- a situation where two things *seem* related, but where, in reality, one does not *cause* the other.

However, if one does the intellectual gymnastics to *believe* that causation exists in an indirect association, then it is entirely possible to "prove" a great many scientific impossibilities.

In this context, it is possible to "prove scientifically" that education makes women infertile. The "science" goes like this: The birth rate among educated women is lower than uneducated women, therefore educated women are less fertile. This illustrates how junk science can look scientifically valid. But in this case, looking more deeply into other factors, you find that educated women are more likely to postpone (or forego) childbearing than uneducated women are. Thus, while lower birth rates are indirectly associated with education, education does not "cause" lower fertility.

This same sort of indirect association *may* account for the links between breast cancer and alcohol. However, since *any* link serves the political agenda of the anti-alcohol groups, they prefer to promote the studies and embellish the data that support their positions and cover-up the data that does not support their agenda.

Indirect associations are fairly common in nature which is why it is so important to take further steps -- to establish a mechanism of how the effect could happen, and to conduct animal studies that could confirm the association.

In this context it it important to note that while anti-alcohol groups promote junk science that "proves" alcohol causes cancer, no biological mechanism has been established for the action and none of the animal studies have shown it to cause cancer.

TWENTY-THREE

Why Do Heart Attacks Happen?

The human heart is a wonderful pump, just a little smaller than a man's clinched fist, that moves about 4,000 gallons of blood per day through your body each day without a rest. A healthy heart will beat more than 2.5 billion times in the average person's lifetime -- unless something goes wrong.

And things go wrong frequently: More than one third of American men and ten percent of American woman can expect to have cardiovascular disease by the age of 60.

More than one third of American men and ten percent of American women can expect to have cardiovascular disease by the age of 60.

What most often goes wrong appears, at first glance, to be a plumbing problem: clogged coronary arteries are unable to supply blood to the heart itself. On a deeper level, the problem is biochemical: the clogs come from an excess of cholesterol.

But on the most basic level, it's usually a lifestyle problem. What we eat and drink, what we choose not to inhale (like tobacco), how we deal with stress and how we exercise all affect the cholesterol which affects the coronary plumbing.

As you'll learn in the next few chapters, the medical treatments that deal with heart disease like a plumbing job for the Roto- Rooter truck are usually doomed to failure without lifestyle changes. Prevention is so much more important than intervention because damaged heart muscle never heals completely. Portions of heart muscles that die form scar tissue that is incapable of contributing to the heart's pumping. Once gone, gone forever.

Plumbing problems

Most heart problems are caused by *ischemia*, insufficient oxygen to the heart, and known as "Ischemic Heart Disease (IHD)" to physicians and researchers. IHD begins when deposits of cholesterol ("plaque")

LIFESTYLE TIP

Moderate alcohol consumption can have an immediate effect on decreasing the blood's tendency to clot in your arteries. Its ability to increase the "good" HDL cholesterol develops more slowly, after continued, regular moderate consumption.

build up in one, or all, of the three coronary arteries that deliver blood to the heart muscle, the *myocardium.* This narrowing of the arteries is known as atherosclerosis or arteriosclerosis.

If the coronary artery blockage is not complete, but is severe enough to cause pain during stress or exercise, the IHD is known as *angina pectoris,* literally "strangling" or "choking in the chest." If the angina episode does not last for very long, the heart muscle may not be damaged. However, if it continues, portions of the muscle could die.

Angina is treated with *vasodilators,* drugs which relax the muscle layer of arteries thereby increasing their diameter and blood flow. The most common vasodilator is nitroglycerin, taken orally or by transdermal skin patch.

Alcohol is also a vasodilator. This property may contribute to the lower coronary death rate among moderate drinkers, although further research is needed.

It's also hypothesized that moderate alcohol consumption may provide some protection against a more dangerous arterial condition which is closely related to angina: spasms.

The coronary artery, like all arteries, has a muscle layer that can contract or relax. This allows your body to regulate blood flow during times of exertion, sending more blood to the working muscles and restricting it to parts of the body (like the digestive organs) which need it less at that time. The muscle walls also affect blood pressure. In fact, without muscle tension in the arteries, your blood pressure would drop to zero and you would die. (This is what happens in anaphylactic shock when sensitive people are exposed to bee stings, penicillin or other allergens).

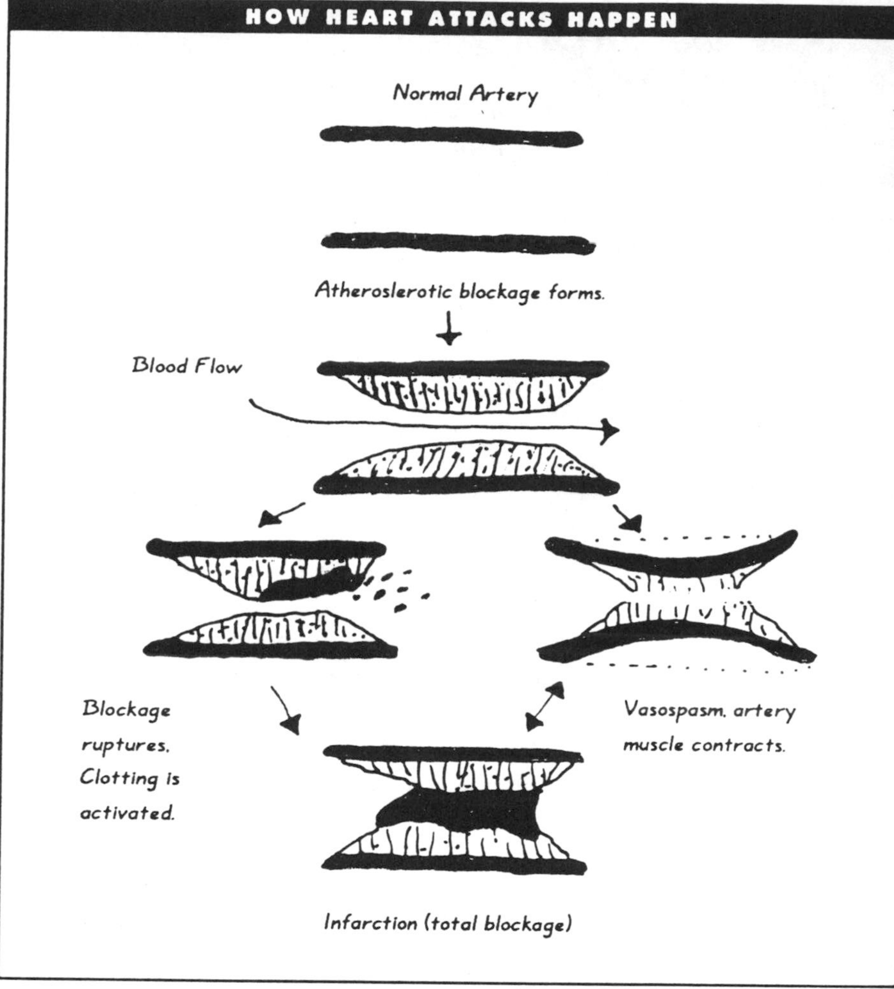

The down side to coronary artery muscles is that they can twitch or spasm just like other muscles. If a healthy artery spasms, little harm may occur. But when they spasm along a section of coronary artery already narrowed by cholesterol plaque, the result could be a complete -- or nearly complete -- cutoff of the blood supply. If the spasms last too long, the heart muscle could be damaged.

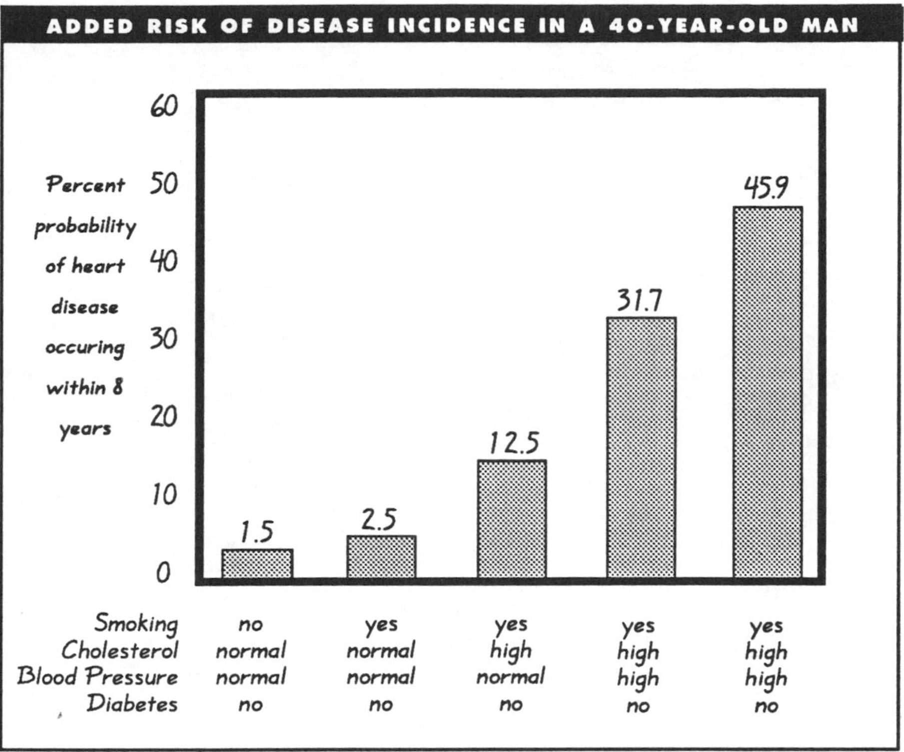

Source: *Framingham Heart Study*

More serious still is an acute *myocardial infarction (MI)*, the classic heart attack which stops its victims in their tracks. The MI is a complete blocking of the coronary artery by a blood clot.

Usually the clot lodges at the point of an existing build-up of cholesterol which has already narrowed the artery. The clot is also called a *thrombus* which is why this kind of heart attack is sometimes called a *coronary thrombosis*.

Sometimes the clot and blockage are caused by part of the cholesterol plaque coming loose from the artery wall and causing the blockage itself. Medical researchers think the process is usually far more complex, involving a combination of other factors.

The process may be caused partly by the tendency of clots to form near artery blockages. This may happen because the blood -- which usually flows smoothly -- becomes turbulent near the cholesterol build-ups. This turbulence (like the eddies that swirl around an obstruction in a stream) may cause damage, to blood platelets or perhaps to the artery walls, which can accelerate clotting. And just as sand and silt tend to accumulate downstream of a river's obstruction, the turbulence may also create the physical condition for a clot to form and grow.

The term "heart attack" is a common but easily misinterpreted term. Physicians usually avoid it because of its imprecision. A heart attack usually encompasses angina, MI, spasms and arrythmias (irregular heart rhythm) although the interpretation may vary from person to person. Because all these conditions cause the heart muscle to suffer from oxygen deprivation, they are all Ischemic Heart Disease. For that reason we will use IHD and heart attack as identical and interchangeable terms in this book.

Platelets are very small cells in the blood, smaller than a red blood cell, which play many key roles in the body, including one in the clotting process. When you receive a cut, many life-saving biochemical processes swing into action to keep you from losing blood. Among these processes, platelets become more "sticky" and begin to clump together to staunch the blood flow. At the same time, a long, stringy protein called *fibrinogen* is produced, tangling itself through the clumping platelets, like reinforcing rods in a concrete dam, making the clot hold together better.

Two other key contributors to fast and efficient clotting are *adrenalin* and *noradrenalin*, hormones produced in times of stress. These hormones evolved as life-saving mechanisms because a person wounded by a saber-tooth tiger or by another person in battle would bleed less and be more likely to survive. These hormones also act as *vasoconstrictors* which narrow the arteries, again preserving blood if wounded.

These defense mechanisms become life-threatening when they happen at the wrong place and time, such as in your coronary arteries.

The actual process may involve turbulence which could help to dislodge part of the plaque; then, the area from which the plaque is dislodged releases chemical messengers that initiate the clotting process. A clot forms, completing the blockage started by the dislodged plaque, and a full-blown myocardial infarction puts the victim just heartbeats away from death and disability.

Research has confirmed that both aspirin and moderate alcohol consumption decrease the stickiness of platelets and their tendency to clot. There are also indications that moderate alcohol consumption may decrease the production of fibrinogen and help dissolve clots once they have formed, a process known as *fibrinolysis.*

Research has confirmed that both aspirin and moderate alcohol consumption decrease the stickiness of platelets and their tendency to clot. There are also indications that moderate alcohol consumption may decrease the production of fibrinogen and help dissolve clots once they have formed, a process known as fibrinolysis.

While all this tells us what goes wrong in the plumbing, and goes some way towards explaining "Why do heart attacks happen?" it just shoves the cause down the line to another question: "Why does cholesterol block arteries?" Read on.

TWENTY-FOUR

Cholesterol And Fats: Jekyll & Hyde Characters

Cholesterol kills.

The reknowned Framingham Heart Study found that the risk of heart disease rises 2 percent for every 1 percent that blood cholesterol levels rise above 150 mg/dl. Dr. William Castelli, M.D., medical director of the Framingham study, says they have not found one heart attack among study group participants whose cholesterol levels are below 150.

> ***The risk of heart disease rises 2 percent for every 1 percent that blood cholesterol levels rise above 150 mg/dl.***

Cholesterol is a Jekyll and Hyde substance.

Arterial blockages by cholesterol kill about half a million people each year, yet cholesterol is in the membranes of every cell. Cholesterol serves as the electrical insulation of nerve cells; the body uses it to make a number of hormones and the crucial Vitamin D.

Cholesterol is so important to your body that your liver can manufacture all you need without you eating even a single gram of it. This is where the problem begins. On its own, the liver will use saturated fats to make the cholesterol it needs. Conversely, the liver filters out the excess cholesterol and excrete its as bile salts. Those salts pass through the gall bladder into the intestinal system where their detergent-like action helps digest other fats and cholesterol. (The cholesterol may not be gone forever since the bile salts are largely reabsorbed from the intestine into the body.)

Cholesterol is like thousands of other beneficial compounds, ranging from aspirin and alcohol to Vitamin A and Zinc. If your body gets too much, thc high concentrations overwhelm the biochemical mechanisms for dealing with it. Suddenly your lifestyle has laid a potentially fatal trap for you.

Scientists think that excess cholesterol is caused by:

LIFESTYLE TIP

Weight loss alone can raise your HDL level by as much as 5 points, according to the National Institutes of Health Multiple Risk Factor Intervention Trial.

Genetics

People have differing abilities to cope with cholesterol. About five percent of the population has levels that remain high despite low intake of cholesterol and fats.

Diet

Most people with elevated cholesterol levels consume too much cholesterol and saturated fat. In addition, these diets are apt to lack fruit, vegetables and other sources of soluble fiber that lower cholesterol levels.

Stress

Studies show that stress tends to raise the overall cholesterol level, with proportionately larger increases for "bad" LDL cholesterol than for "good" HDL.

Lack of Exercise

Moderate exercise can raise your HDL levels and help lower overall cholesterol levels. It is not clear whether the lower level is due directly to the exercise or to its stress-reducing effect.

Obviously, this book can't do anything about your genetic make-up. If you're the 1-in-20 person whose cholesterol level is genetically unable to respond to lifestyle changes, you need to see your physician to discuss other options such as drug therapy. But for the rest of the population, diet, stress reduction and exercise can all help save your life.

What The Heck Is Cholesterol?

Cholesterol is a waxy chemical with a complex molecular ring structure that, by itself, is insoluble in blood.

CHOLESTEROL

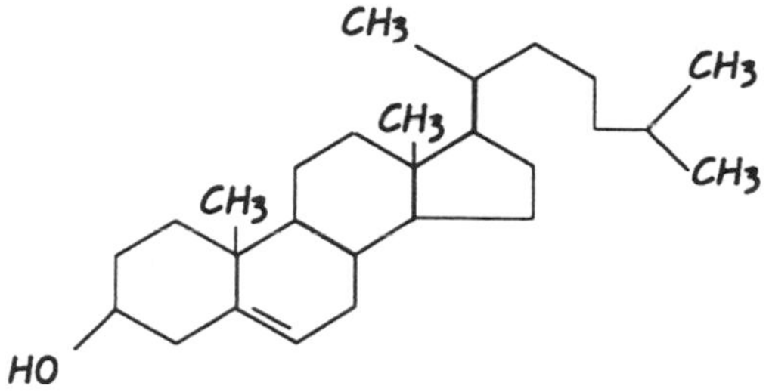

CH_3 CH_3 CH_3 CH_3 CH_3 HO

Because of this insolubility, cholesterol needs a blood-soluble compound to transport it through the body. The suitable vehicle is another molecule called *lipoprotein.* This is a disk- shaped molecule with a fat (lipo) portion, that attaches to the cholesterol, and a protein portion that surrounds the cholesterol and makes the whole package soluble in your water-based blood. In one sense, the cholesterol molecule rides inside the lipoprotein like an astronaut in a hockey-puck-shaped space capsule.

Lipoproteins are a vital part of the cholesterol equation. You've seen the reference to "good" HDL and "bad" LDL cholesterol. Well, you've been tricked, in a small way, for the sake of explaining a complex biochemical situation. Cholesterol is the same molecule regardless of whether it's riding in an HDL or an LDL capsule. But how the lipoprotein capsule operates determines whether the cholesterol is "good" or "bad."

Blood lipoproteins are very specialized. LDL carries cholesterol from the liver to the body's cells; HDL carries excess cholesterol from the cells to the liver.

When an LDL gets to a cell that needs cholesterol, it unloads its cholesterol molecule. When all your cells have enough cholesterol, it's another story. The LDL particles circulate continuously through the blood where a finite number of them bind with LDL receptors, primarily in the liver. Binding with an LDL receptor removes the cholesterol from

LIFESTYLE TIP

Read food labels carefully to avoid hidden sources of saturated fats that raise your cholesterol levels. They're frequently found in store-bought cookies, crackers, cake and pastry mixes and many snack foods. This is one more reason to avoid processed "techno-foods."

the blood. Genetic variations in the number of LDL receptors may account for our ability to handle cholesterol.

When the LDL receptors are saturated, the LDLs circulate through the blood and, through a complicated series of biochemical steps, eventually end up dumping their cholesterol loads in your arteries. Atherosclerosis begins.

High LDL levels work against you in another way. Research has shown that high LDL levels actually **decrease** the number of LDL receptors, thus making a bad situation worse. Saturated fats are another double whammy. They decrease LDL receptor activity **and** increase LDL levels. When things go wrong, they can go wrong big time.

On the other hand, HDL circulates through the blood like a taxi cruising for a cholesterol fare to take back to the liver, which converts it to bile salts. More HDL circulating means more cholesterol gets scavenged from your system and returned to the liver for a safe exit.

Scientists still don't know if HDL is the prime mover in cholesterol removal or if some other hidden factor actually prompts the HDL to perform its job. Like so many other things, we know that high concentrations of HDLs are associated with a decreased risk of heart disease and we know **how** HDLs perform this service. Science just doesn't know yet **why** it works. When we know the **why** we may begin to understand how moderate alcohol consumption and other factors increase HDLs.

Today, science does know that lowering overall cholesterol is important to decreasing heart attack risk. Further, it's important to have as high a proportion of HDL as possible.

Dr. Meir Stampfer of Harvard Medical School found in a 1988 study that a **1-point increase in HDL produced about a 7 percent reduction in heart attack risk.**

People who measure only their total cholesterol are missing a crucial part of their health equation. A good overall target for which to aim is 150 but the ratio of total cholesterol to HDL is equally important.

The Framingham study indicates that a ratio of 5:1 (total cholesterol:HDL) puts men at an "average" risk of heart attack; 4:1 for women. This ratio would be found in someone with a total cholesterol level of 180 in which LDL measured 150 and HDL, 30.

While 180 is significantly below the 200 level for which most people strive, another person with the same total cholesterol level would be at higher risk if the HDL measured only 15 -- a ratio of 11:1.

As you can see, raising or lowering the HDL level can dramatically alter the ratio. A ratio of 3:1 cuts your risk to less than half of the average; your risk doubles at 9.5:1. People with ratios of more than 23:1 triple their heart attack risk.

Zapping Chylomicron Invaders From The Triglyceride Nebula

Like cholesterol, fats (triglycerides) are substances your body can't do without, but which can kill you if you eat too

HDL can be divided into two major sub-categories, HDL2 and HDL3. Following the discovery that alcohol consumption increased HDL levels, some researchers -- particularly those funded by anti-alcohol organizations -- denigrated the cardio-protective effects. These studies asserted that only HDL2 was cardio-protective and that alcohol raised the HDL3 component. More recent research has shown that* both *types of HDL are cardio- protective, thus proving at least one mechanism by which alcohol consumption can reduce the risk of heart disease.

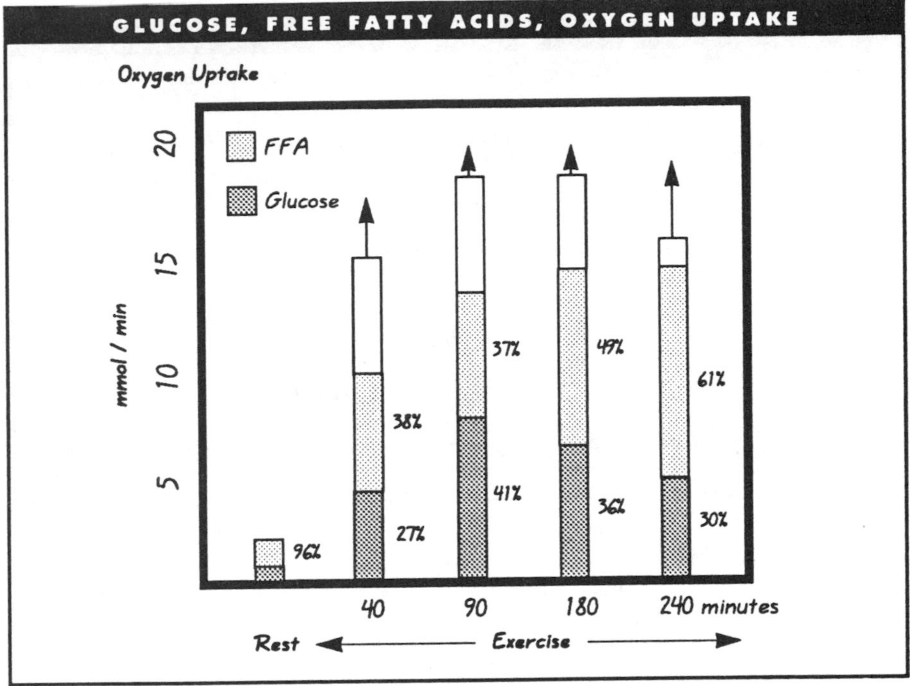

Source: Wahren et. al. Diabetologia. 1978

much. Sustained high blood concentrations of fat, *hyperlipidemia*, are suspected of being one of the factors that damage artery walls and promote atherosclerosis.

But fats are also necessary for cell growth, for the body's synthesis of needed chemicals and for energy. During sustained exercise, free fatty acids provide 40 to 60 percent of the affected muscle's energy. The longer the exercise, the more the muscles rely on fatty acids. In fact, your longest-exercising muscle -- the heart -- relies almost exclusively on free fatty acids (FFAs) for its energy.

Like cholesterol, fats are not soluble in your water-based blood; they need specialized transport vehicles to get them from one place in your body to another. Those transport vehicles are also lipoproteins. Both VLDL (very low density lipoprotein) and *chylomicrons* deal with triglyceride transport.

A TRYGLYCERIDE

$$\text{Glycerol} \left\{ \begin{array}{l} CH_2 - O - \overset{O}{\overset{\bullet}{C}} - R \\ CH \ \ - O - \overset{O}{\overset{\bullet}{C}} - R \\ CH_2 - O - \overset{O}{\overset{\bullet}{C}} - R \end{array} \right.$$

▲ *fatty acid*

The "R" represents fatty acids chemically bound to the glycerol backbone of the triglyceride.

VLDLs contain some cholesterol but primarily transport triglycerides to adipose tissue for storage as fat. VLDL can be converted into LDL; in a blood test it is counted as part of the LDLs.

Chylomicrons primarily move fat from the intestine to the liver. From there it is either converted to VLDLs for transportation to love handles and double chins or stored as fat in the liver itself.

Chylomicrons are processed rapidly and are mostly gone within 9 to 15 hours after you eat the mealtime fats that prompted their formation. Blood for triglyceride tests is usually drawn first thing in the morning before you have had anything to eat (and nothing since dinner the evening before -- a 12- to 15-hour fasting interval). That's so the VLDL triglyceride levels will not have been altered by chylomicron concentrations.

Like most people, you may be confused by the apparently inconsistent use of the words: fat, oil, fatty acids, triglycerides. The differences and similarities are easy to understand. Fats and oils are both triglycerides; the only difference is that at room temperature fats tend to be solids and oils tend to be liquids. For most non-technical purposes, fat, oil and triglyceride can be used interchangeably.

COMPARISON OF THE STRUCTURE OF FOUR FATTY ACIDS

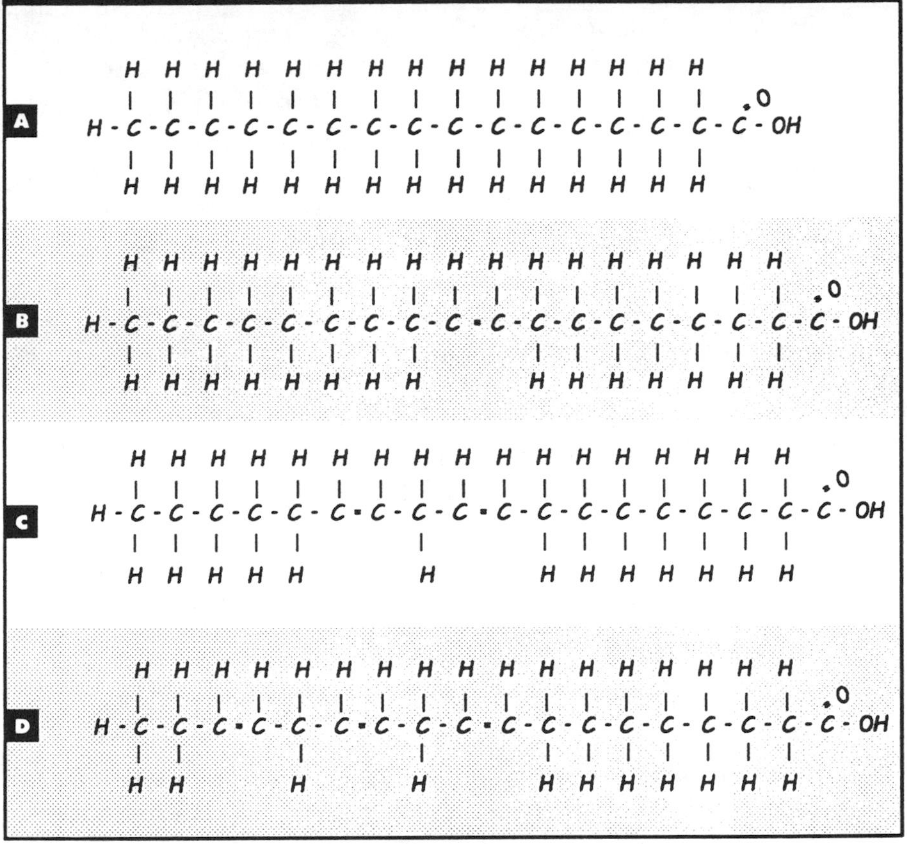

A

```
    H   H   H   H   H   H   H   H   H   H   H   H   H   H
    |   |   |   |   |   |   |   |   |   |   |   |   |   |   .O
H - C - C - C - C - C - C - C - C - C - C - C - C - C - C - C - OH
    |   |   |   |   |   |   |   |   |   |   |   |   |   |
    H   H   H   H   H   H   H   H   H   H   H   H   H   H
```

B

```
    H   H   H   H   H   H   H   H   H   H   H   H   H   H   H   H   H
    |   |   |   |   |   |   |   |   |   |   |   |   |   |   |   |   |   .O
H - C - C - C - C - C - C - C - C - C ▪ C - C - C - C - C - C - C - C - C - OH
    |   |   |   |   |   |   |   |           |   |   |   |   |   |   |
    H   H   H   H   H   H   H   H           H   H   H   H   H   H   H
```

C

```
    H   H   H   H   H   H   H   H   H   H   H   H   H   H   H   H   H
    |   |   |   |   |   |   |   |   |   |   |   |   |   |   |   |   |   .O
H - C - C - C - C - C - C ▪ C - C - C ▪ C - C - C - C - C - C - C - C - C - OH
    |   |   |   |   |           |           |   |   |   |   |   |   |
    H   H   H   H   H           H           H   H   H   H   H   H   H
```

D

```
    H   H   H   H   H   H   H   H   H   H   H   H   H   H   H   H   H
    |   |   |   |   |   |   |   |   |   |   |   |   |   |   |   |   |   .O
H - C - C - C ▪ C - C - C ▪ C - C - C ▪ C - C - C - C - C - C - C - C - C - OH
    |   |           |           |           |   |   |   |   |   |   |
    H   H           H           H           H   H   H   H   H   H   H
```

a) palmitic, b) oleic, c) linoleic, and d) linoleic acids

Triglycerides are molecules composed of three (thus the "tri") fatty acids bound to a glycerol (thus the "glyceride") molecule.

(To confuse the layperson even more, an international scientific nomenclature commission has ruled that the word *triacylgylcerol* is more scientifically correct than triglyceride. You may start seeing this new word in magazines and newspapers.)

The glycerol (also known as glycerine) is identical in all triglycerides (fats). But what makes a fat "good" or "bad" for your health depends on which three fatty acids are hooked up to it.

The bad fatty acids are those which have the maximum number of hydrogen atoms attached to them -- they are "saturated". Saturated fats tend to raise your cholesterol level.

Unsaturated fatty acids have slightly fewer calories than saturated fat since they have fewer hydrogen atoms to be oxidized during metabolism.

Conversely, fatty acids whose molecules do not have all the hydrogen possible are known as "unsaturated." Monounsaturated fats contain molecules that are only one hydrogen short of saturation while polyunsaturated fatty acids lack two or more hydrogen atoms.

Polyunsaturated fats are better than saturated for decreasing heart disease risk, but some studies have indicated that a diet high in polyunsaturated fats may increase the risk of cancer and also lower HDL levels. Monounsaturated fats (like olive and canola oils) are most effective at increasing good HDLs and do not have an associated increase in cancer risk.

A glycerol can have two or three different kinds of fatty acids hooked up to it or they can all be the same. In fact, fats and oils are all mixtures of saturated, mono- and polyunsaturated fatty acids. Olive oil, for instance, is known as "heart healthy" because it contains more monounsaturated fatty acids (77 percent) than any other dietary oils. But even olive oil contains saturated fatty acids (14 percent) and polyunsaturated fatty acids (9 percent). By contrast, beef fat is 50 percent saturated fatty acid, 42 percent monounsaturated and 4 percent polyunsaturated. But the kings of saturation are tropical oils. Coconut oil is 86 percent saturated and palm kernel, 81 percent.

Food technologists, however, are rarely content with the foods that nature has provided; oils are no exception. Food manufacturers will often put unsaturated vegetable oils through a chemical process known as "hydrogenation" that adds hydrogen to the fat molecule. While this

> **LIFESTYLE TIP**
>
> ***When you see "hydrogenated vegetable oil" on a product's list of ingredients, remember that this is just another name for "saturated fat," and can be just as bad for you. Healthy eating demands that you restrict your intake of these foods.***

increases shelf life and changes the texture of the resulting fat or oil, it also robs the formerly unsaturated oil of some of its health benefits. Margarine and all-vegetable lard are two examples of partially hydrogenated vegetable oils. These were among the earliest techno-foods..

A Healthy Fish Story

There was much to-do several years ago about the cardio- protective nature of oils from salmon and other cold-water fish. Those oils contain a high concentration of omega-3 polyunsaturated fatty acids.

Lab research suggests that omega-3 fatty acids don't seem to affect cholesterol levels. In fact, participants in one lab study who ate about 1 tablespoon of fish oil per day actually increased their LDLs. These types of fish oils, however, do seem to help prevent atherosclerosis by decreasing the tendency of white blood cells called *monocytes* to stick to artery walls. However, little more is known, including whether you get the same protective effect by taking pill supplements containing

AN OMEGA-3 FATTY ACID: EICOSAPENTAENOIC ACID

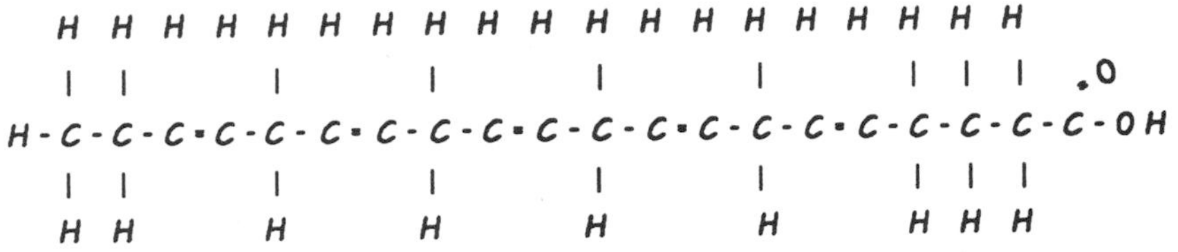

```
  H H H H H H H H H H H H H H H H H H H
  | |   |   |   |   |   | | |  .O
H-C-C-C•C-C-C•C-C-C•C-C-C•C-C-C•C-C-C-C-C-OH
  | |   |   |   |   |   | | |
  H H   H   H   H   H   H H H
```

▲ *Omega end of the fatty acid*

OMEGA-3 FATTY ACIDS IN FISH

	GRAMS		GRAMS
Sardines (Norwegian)	5.1	Bluefish	1.2
Sockeye salmon	2.7	Pacific Mackerel	1.1
Atlantic mackerel	2.5	Striped bass	0.8
King salmon	1.9	Yellowfin tuna	0.6
Herring	1.7	Pollock	0.5
Lake trout	1.4	Brook trout	0.4
Albacore tuna	1.3	Yellow perch	0.3
Halibut	1.3	Catfish	0.2

omega-3 fatty acids. Eating lots of salmon is more fun, but grill it or use olive oil in the preparation; butter only ruins the health effect. And don't bother with fish oil capsules. Just eat lots of fish instead. The *New England Journal of Medicine* has reported that men who daily ate an average of 30 grams (slightly more than one ounce) of fish rich in omega-3 fatty acids cut their heart attack risk in half -- that's just 7 ounces per week.

Cholesterol is measured in milligrams per deciliter of blood (abbreviated mg/dl). A deciliter is one-tenth of a liter and a liter is slightly smaller than a quart. A milligram is one- thousandth of a gram and there are 454 grams in a pound. When people refer to their cholesterol as "225" or "178" they are referring to mg/dl.

TARGET CHOLESTEROL LEVELS

	DESIRABLE less than	BORDERLINE HIGH less than	HIGH RISK greater than
Total Cholesterol	200	240	240
LDL-cholesterol	130	160	160

Source: U.S. Dept. of Health $ Human Services

To Think About

New beverage specific consumption data show wine is primarily consumed with meals in a family setting and *"usually deemed appropriate in integrative, social enjoyment enhancing situations."* Pittman, D., and Klein, H., "Perceived Consequences Associated With the Use of Beer, Wine, Distilled Spirits, and Wine Coolers." International Journal of Addiction, Vol. 25, p. 19, 1989.

TWENTY-FIVE

Why Do Coronary Arteries Clog Up?

Medical science knows much about the mechanical aspects of heart disease and heart attacks. We know a fair amount about cholesterol, triglycerides and fatty acids.

But exactly how the body's vital substances turn against it is somewhat sketchier. In the last two chapters, the material has been mostly scientific **fact**. This chapter will deal more with **hypothesis** -- educated theories that are backed up by a body of research, but which have not yet been proven conclusively.

What's A Clot?

Contrary to popular belief, coronary artery blockages are not simple rubbish heaps of cholesterol. Instead, they are complicated structures composed of connective tissue, cholesterol, muscle cells from the artery wall, and other tissues. In fact, this mass, called an *atherosclerotic lesion* by physicians, loosely resembles a partially healed wound on other parts of the body.

Coronary arteries undergo characteristic changes in people and other mammals fed a diet high in fat and cholesterol.

Medical research shows that coronary arteries undergo characteristic changes in people and other mammals fed a diet high in fat and cholesterol. The first stage, scientists believe, is an injury to the *intima*, the inner lining of the artery.

The atherosclerotic process begins when white blood cells, known as *monocytes*, invade the artery wall and embed themselves just inside the first layer of cells.

Monocytes play a role in the body's immune system and can activate other immune defenses when they sense an infection. A Monocyte is also capable of transforming itself into an amoeba- like scavenger cell known as a *macrophage* that attacks bacteria and other foreign objects by surrounding them (like the B-movie Blob did to its larger victims).

Atherosclerosis is a process of chronic irritation which steadily develops over decades. Unless the substance that triggers the irritation is removed, the lesion grows and grows until it kills.

Monocytes collect near injuries (such as a cut finger) and are the majority of cells contained in the pus that collects around an infection or injury.

This early involvement of monocytes is one of the strongest clues that atherosclerosis begins with some sort of injury to the artery wall.

Once embedded in the artery wall, the monocytes transform themselves into macrophages which then consume so much cholesterol they resemble fat-filled foam. This early stage of atherosclerosis, present in most people by the end of their 30s, forms fatty streaks in the artery walls which don't appear to be harmful by themselves.

But, as the foamy macrophages gorge on cholesterol, they expand and break through the thin inner layer of artery wall cells and become exposed to the blood. The exposed macrophages attract another part of the blood system -- platelets. The platelets then release a number of proteins, some of which promote the growth of the artery's muscle cells.

The new artery muscle cells synthesize connective tissues (hard, leathery substances which are the main components of ligaments, tendons and scar tissue) that make the lesion more permanent.

The new artery muscle cells absorb LDL cholesterol at much higher rates than normal intima cells. Cellular debris from cells that have died are also embedded in this matrix of new muscle cells, cholesterol particles and connective tissue.

Atherosclerosis is a process of chronic irritation which steadily develops over decades. Unless the substance that triggers the irritation is removed, the lesion grows and grows until it kills.

Trigger factors

Unfortunately, there seems to be no shortage of substances that can injure an artery wall. Some of the most important are:

- high levels of fat and cholesterol,
- tobacco,
- high blood pressure,
- stress,
- being male or post-menopausal female and
- glucose intolerance/high insulin levels (diabetes or borderline diabetes).

LIFESTYLE TIP

Every 1 percent reduction in blood cholesterol levels reduces heart attack risk by nearly 2 percent.

High levels of fat and cholesterol

Fat and cholesterol don't just form part of the atherosclerotic lesion; they may actually help cause the injury that triggered it in the first place.

The LDL, VLDL, and chylomicron molecules themselves may actually irritate artery walls, much like a minor abrasion on the skin. It's not known for sure what causes the irritation, but scientists have hypothesized that it might come from the high chemical reactivity of the double-bonded oxygen atom on the end of every fatty acid. This end of the fatty acid is usually the one exposed since it is the most soluble in the blood. In theory, the active oxygen atom could reach out and steal a hydrogen atom from surrounding tissues, a process known as *oxidation.* If done millions or billions of times, the damage grows serious.

Oxidation's contribution to atherosclerosis is a subject of much hypothesizing. In addition to the possible involvement of the oxygen on the fatty acid chain, many other chemicals -- known as *free radicals* -- can cause similar damage. The science of free radicals and their role in human health is still somewhat embryonic. But it's suspected that some may come directly from harmful substances we eat or breath and

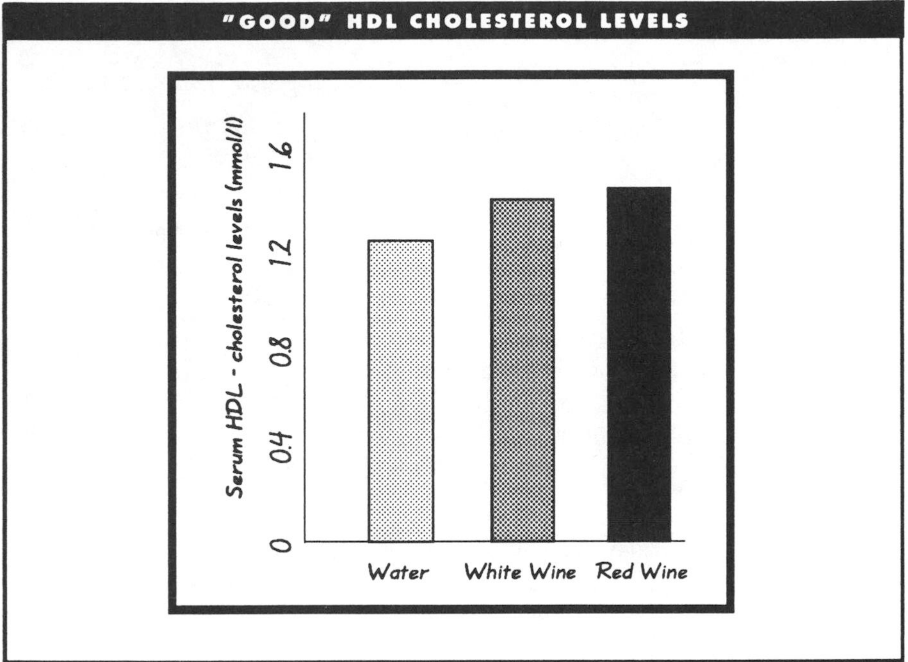

Source: Jour. Applied Cardiology. 1990. Vol. 5

others may come from the metabolism of fat and other food components.

In addition to a role in atherosclerosis, oxidants/free radicals are suspected of playing a role in cancer and some genetic defects.

Research has shown that the remnants of lipoproteins, left over after the contents have been delivered, may help cause atherosclerosis. Although the exact mechanism is not yet fully known, these fragments may form oxidizing free radicals. In addition, they may contribute to cholesterol deposits in an artery. Even though VLDLs and chylomicrons primarily transport triglycerides, they both contain cholesterol (as much as 45 percent in some VLDLs) which may remain with the remnant and contribute to artery lesions. Other research suggests that free radicals may damage LDL molecules in a way that makes them more likely to be deposited at lesion sites.

The researchers who manage to prove a unified theory on oxidants and heart disease will most likely find themselves on an airplane to Stockholm to pick up their Nobel Prize.

Tobacco

Long recognized as the leading cause of lung cancer, tobacco smoking causes more deaths from heart attack than cancer. Nicotine is a vasoconstrictor which raises blood pressure and decreases the blood supply to the heart and brain. This vasoconstriction alone can precipitate a stroke or heart attack.

LIFESTYLE TIP

"Sudden death is the most frequent clinical event associated with cigarette smoking." -- *Textbook of Medicine,* ***Beeson, McDermott & Wyngaarden***

But cigarettes may also injure arteries. In addition to nicotine, cigarette smoke is a potent stew of toxic chemicals ranging from formaldehyde to cyanide. These poisons can kill cells in the artery walls and pave the way for atherosclerosis. In addition, components of cigarette smoking:

- ♥ accelerate the clotting process;
- ♥ may cause cardiac rhythm problems,(arrythmias) and
- ♥ are allergenic to many people.

High Blood Pressure (Hypertension)

Water pipes crack and burst under too much pressure. High blood pressure, in most cases, has a far less dramatic effect, but there are indications that raising blood pressure may cause minute fissures in the artery wall, providing a site for a lesion to begin. Other research indicates that the injuries from high blood pressure may also come from turbulence in specific areas of an artery.

High blood pressure (above 160/95) can increase risks dramatically. For example, an otherwise healthy 35-year-old man with a blood pressure of 142/90 has twice the chance of dying from a heart attack within 20 years than if his blood pressure were 120/80. A level of 152/95 increases the chance to 2.5 times.

Stress

Stress can raise blood pressure by constricting arteries; it also makes blood more likely to clot. In addition, the adrenalin produced while people are under stress mobilizes the body's fat stores and raises the blood levels of free fatty acids (FFAs) to provide muscle energy. If, as some hypothesize, the oxygen molecule is an oxidant, chronic high levels of stress-induced FFAs may contribute to the formation of atherosclerotic lesions.

Finally, stress actually raises LDL cholesterol levels. Studies of tax accountants found steady increases in LDL leading up to and peaking around April 15. Levels steadily eased off afterwards.

LIFESTYLE TIP

The American Heart Association estimates that passive smoking (non-smokers who inhale cigarette toxins from smokers) kills 53,000 people per year including 37,000 from heart attacks. Avoiding cigarette smoke is not just a matter of avoiding the smell, it's a matter of life and death for non-smokers.

Being Male, Or A Post-Menopausal Female

While pre-menopausal heart disease in women has increased in the past 20 years (due primarily to increases in cigarette smoking and job stress), women under 60 still have less than one-third the risk (one woman in 10) of having a heart attack as men of the same age (one man in three).

Estrogen, it seems, increases HDLs while testosterone reduces it. From adolescence on, men have a 10 to 20 percent lower HDL than women and about 10 percent higher LDL.

Moderate consumption of alcohol plays a role in this sex-related mechanism. A 1992 study at the University of Pittsburgh found that post-menopausal women who were moderate alcohol consumers had a lower coronary death rate than abstainers or heavy drinkers, primarily because of increased levels of *estradiol* (one of the female sex hormones). The research indicated that alcohol may contribute by helping to change androgen (male sex hormones) into estradiol. It's known that female hormones are found in very low levels in men and male hormones in women. While no research yet exists on the effect of alcohol on male estrogen levels, this might offer one possible mechanism for alcohol's cardio-protective effect.

Post-menopausal women who were moderate alcohol consumers a lower coronary death rate than abstainers or heavy drinkers, primarily because of increased levels of estradiol (one of the female sex hormones).

Glucose Intolerance

Physicians have known for decades that people suffering from diabetes have astronomically high risks of heart disease; uncontrolled diabetes almost always leads to blood vessel damage and heart disease.

Diabetes works its evil because another vital substance, *glucose* becomes damaging once its concentration in the blood rises too high. Glucose is a simple sugar which is used for energy by most body cells. But when concentrations remain high (150 mg/dl) for long periods, they damage the tiniest of arteries, *arterioles*, which supply blood directly to the tissues. This causes the poor circulation which many diabetics first experience in their hands and feet; it also scars and blocks coronary arterioles.

Diabetes is characterized primarily by the body's inability to produce enough insulin which helps the body metabolize glucose and also affects the storage and metabolism of fatty acids.

While low insulin levels allow glucose to build up in the blood, high levels can be equally detrimental. Insulin stimulates the production of fatty acids (from glucose and similar compounds) which then increases blood triglyceride levels as VLDL molecules transport the new fat to storage in adipose cells. While the fat deposited under your waist is no longer circulating in the blood, the remnants of the VLDLs continue along, contributing their atherosclerotic damage.

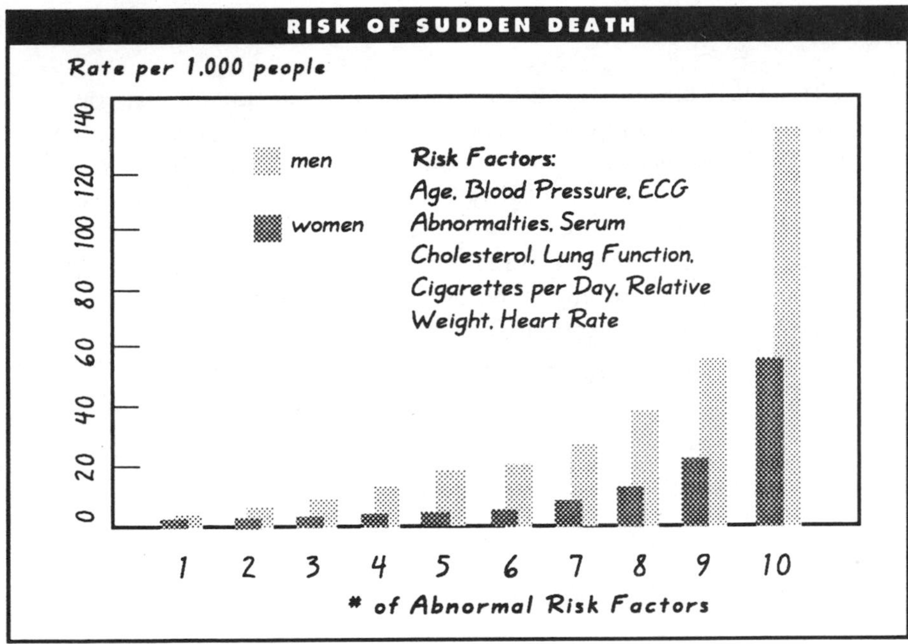

Source: Framingham Heart Study

The January 1992 issue of the *British Medical Journal* confirmed that women who drink alcohol moderately have the same reduced heart disease risks as men. But the study also found that while these women had elevated HDLs and lower levels of triglycerides and LDLs, they also had lower insulin levels (without suffering from the glucose intolerance found in diabetics).

This research supports the hypothesis that alcohol, particularly when consumed moderately with meals, tends to moderate insulin levels. It keeps them from hitting harmful peaks but without impairing the body's ability to handle glucose.

In addition, soluble fiber, found in fresh fruits and vegetables as well as in beans and oat bran, seems to help diabetics maintain stable glucose levels. This may also contribute to heart health in non-diabetics as well.

Obesity

The role of obesity is somewhat confused. While most obese people have elevated fat and cholesterol levels, high-blood pressure and an increased incidence of diabetes, research shows that when these factors are removed, excess weight by itself has little relationship to increased risk of heart disease. (*Textbook of Medicine*, Beeson, McDermott & Wyngaarden, 15th edition, p.1221). Studies have shown that weight loss in people with high cholesterol levels can reduce overall cholesterol and increase HDLs.

Sidebar Thirteen

Strokes of Misfortune

Strokes come in two varieties, hemorrhagic (bleeding) and occlusive (blocking).

The bleeding variety occurs when a blood vessel in the brain ruptures. They can be prompted by high blood pressure, aneurysms or by substances that interfere with clotting like aspirin or large doses of alcohol. The blocking variety is analogous to a heart attack in the brain where artery blockage occurs.

Studies show that moderate alcohol consumption results in a very small (some studies say no) effect on the hemorrhagic variety and may possibly decrease the occlusive variety which occurs about 10 times more frequently.

A recent study, conducted by a team led by Dr. Arthur L. Klatsky, M.D., at the Kaiser Permanente Medical Center in Oakland, Calif. (*Stroke*, 1989) concluded that, "Daily consumption of three or more drinks, but not lighter drinking was related to higher hospitalization rates for hemorrhagic cerebrovascular disease."

Their data indicated that people who consumed one to two drinks per day had a 0.75 relative risk of being hospitalized for hemorrhagic stroke compared to abstainers (RR = 1.00). Those drinking three or more drinks per day had a relative risk of 1.38.

The Klatsky study also found an indication that moderate alcohol consumption offered some protection against occlusive strokes. Their data indicated that people consuming one to two drinks per day had a relative risk of occlusive stroke of 0.37 compared with abstainers (RR = 1.00). People consuming three or more drinks per day had a relative risk of 0.50.

The Klatsky paper cautions that, "A single study cannot establish an inverse relation between alcohol use and cerebrovascular disease." Since then, several other studies have shown a similar relationship.

The similarity between ischemic heart disease and occlusive strokes makes it plausible that this inverse relationship will continue to be confirmed by future studies.

TWENTY-SIX

Cirrhosis And Alcohol

Your liver is a spongy, jack-of-all-trades organ that performs more than 1,500 chemical functions vital to life. Among those many functions, this brown, three to four pound abdominal organic chemistry factory:

- ♥ detoxifies poisons, both those produced by the body and those from outside,
- ♥ filters bacteria from the blood,
- ♥ regulates fat metabolism,
- ♥ stores and manufactures vitamins,
- ♥ regulates and manufactures cholesterol and fats,
- ♥ synthesizes proteins,
- ♥ maintains the body's water and salt balance,
- ♥ secretes bile for the digestion of fat,
- ♥ stores energy (in the form of glycogen),
- ♥ helps regulate overall body metabolism,
- ♥ transforms the highly toxic ammonia (produced by exercise and by metabolism of proteins) into urea which is eliminated in the urine,
- ♥ manufactures lipoproteins for fat and cholesterol transport and
- ♥ metabolizes alcohol.

> ***There is no evidence that liver injury will occur in healthy men who consume fewer than four drinks per day and healthy women who daily consume fewer than three drinks.***

Because of its vital functions, the liver receives about 25 percent of the heart's output, which forces the blood through the liver's billions of microscopic channels.

Prohibition-era activists, like modern-day anti-alcohol activists, exaggerated the threat to ordinary drinkers from cirrhosis, to scare them away from alcohol.

What Is Cirrhosis?

Cirrhosis is a condition in which the liver's active cells are replaced by fibrous scar tissue which lacks the ability to perform any of the hundreds of required chemical functions. When enough liver cells are replaced by scar tissue, you die.

The relationship between alcohol consumption and cirrhosis of the liver, a relatively rare condition, has been a problematic one for centuries. Prohibition-era activists, like modern-day anti-alcohol activists, exaggerated the threat to ordinary drinkers from cirrhosis, to scare them away from alcohol. But the fact is that most alcoholics will **not** get cirrhosis and many cirrhosis victims are people who have never drunk alcohol.

While alcohol abusers are more likely to suffer from cirrhosis than moderate drinkers (if you drink 14 drinks per day for 33 years, you have an 80 percent chance of getting it), the exact mechanisms of what

ALCHOHOL, WINE & DISEASE

COUNTRY	ALL CAUSES	CANCER	CARDIO VASCULAR	CIRR-HOSIS	VIOLENT DEATH	WINE CONSUMPTION	TOTAL ALCOHOL**
	(Death rate per 100.000)						
JAPAN	838	228	289	21	105	.27	6.3
GREECE	933	215	421	14	97	7.90	5.6
FRANCE	1007	305	310	31	158	19.55	13.3
USA	1060	246	464	17	137	2.24	7.6
IRELAND	1213	305	595	10	108	.95	6.1

*Wine Consumption in Gallons

** Total Alcohol Consumption in Liters of Pure Alcohol

Source: Adapted From "World Health Statistics Annual". WHO. 1989.

causes it are still unclear. Indeed, there is no evidence that liver injury will occur in healthy men who consume fewer than four drinks per day and healthy women who daily consume fewer than three drinks.

Not A Major Problem

While it is an important cause of illness and death, cirrhosis is not the major public health problem posed by coronary artery disease. In the United States (where annual per capita alcohol consumption is about 7.6 liters), the World Health Organization's 1989 *World Health Statistics Annual* found that the death rate from cirrhosis of the liver was 17 per 100,000 while cardiovascular disease killed 464 per 100,000. By contrast, the same study shows France (where per capita alcohol consumption is about 13 liters) with almost double the cirrhosis rate -- 31 per 100,000 -- but with cardiovascular rates at only 310 per 100,000.

If the U.S. wine consumption and death rates were normalized with those of France, 7 more people per 100,000 (the half associated with alcohol) would die of cirrhosis, but 161 fewer people would die of cardiovascular disease. This is a net savings of 151 people who would live longer in order to die later of something else (for, after all, the death rate is eventually 100 percent).

On the face of it, this seems to show a direct, linear relationship between alcohol consumption and cirrhosis. But you can't make a decision based on just two points on a graph. Consider Japan whose per capita alcohol consumption is a bit lower than the United States at 6.3 liters and whose cirrhosis rate is 25 percent higher at 21 per 100,000. Ireland which also consumes about the same amount, 6.1 liters, has a cirrhosis rate less than one-fourth of the United States, 4 per 100,000.

Some alcohol-control advocacy groups assert that cirrhosis rates are artificially lower in some countries because the accuracy of diagnoses of the causes of death varies from country to country. No scientific evidence exists to prove such claims.

"There are data, in fact, to suggest that ethanol [the main form of alcohol in beverages], per se, is not the cause of liver disease in abusers of alcohol,"— Dr. David Zakim, M.D.

However, health statistics from numerous Western countries, including the U.S., indicate that only a fraction of the cirrhosis deaths can be attributed to alcohol consumption.

Dr. David Zakim, M.D., indicates that approximately half of cirrhosis deaths are associated with alcohol.

Taking this into account and using the WHO's death rate numbers, it is not hard to see that if the U.S. wine consumption and death rates were normalized with those of France, 7 more people per 100,000 (the half associated with alcohol) would die of cirrhosis, but 161 fewer people would die of cardiovascular disease. This is a net savings of 151 people who would live longer in order to die later of something else (for, after all, the death rate is eventually 100 percent).

In fact the statistics also hide a striking pattern in the French cirrhosis rates. Dr. Serge Renaud said that INSERM studied the rates on a regional basis and found the highest cirrhosis rates (50 to 100 per 100,000) in areas like those in the northern regions of Alsace and Lorraine which have the highest consumption of beer and spirits.

However, locales with the highest wine consumption, such as Provence, (which consume less beer and spirits), had the lowest cirrhosis rates -- 7 to 14 per 100,000 -- putting them even lower than the U.S.

Alcohol Alone May Not Cause Cirrhosis

"There are data, in fact, to suggest that ethanol [the main form of alcohol in beverages], per se, is not the cause of liver disease in abusers of alcohol," wrote Dr. David Zakim, M.D., author of "Pathophysiology of Liver Disease" published in the medical textbook, *Pathophysiology: The Biological Principles of Disease.* Dr. Zakim writes about two "well-controlled" studies which found that large doses of ethanol administered to hospitalized abusers as a way to ease the rigors of recovery, "did not impede clinical and laboratory recovery from decompensated alcohol-induced liver disease in patients eating a normal hospital diet."

LIFESTYLE TIP

Eating food while drinking alcohol is healthier in two ways: (1) it slows down absorption, preventing quick, large peaks in blood alcohol level and (2) helps metabolize alcohol faster.

Dr. Zakim, who is the Vincent Astor Distinguished Professor of Medicine at the Cornell University Medical College, Professor of Cell Biology at the Cornell University Graduate School of Medical Sciences and Director of the New York Hospital Division of Digestive Diseases, writes that, "**Neither malnutrition nor ethanol ingestion causes serious liver disease, yet abuse of ethanol plus malnutrition produces liver disease in some patients.** The cirrhogenic potential of ethanol is due to interactions with environmental factors, presumably with serious forms of liver disease requiring, in addition, a **susceptible host** [emphasis added] ... The best evidence available indicates that ethanol alone does not produce liver disease."

This uncertain relationship, however, should not be taken as a carte blanche to abuse alcohol since abuse **does** put you in a higher risk category.

Alcohol Metabolism

The liver is the focus of medical research into the effects, both beneficial and harmful, of alcohol. The liver metabolizes alcohol and is the focus of cholesterol and fat synthesis, transport and regulation.

Alcohol in wine, beer and spirits is absorbed through the membranes of the mouth and the esophagus, but mostly from the stomach and intestines. The speed with which it is absorbed varies with the type of alcoholic beverage: the higher the alcohol concentration, the faster it is absorbed. Straight spirits are absorbed faster than wine and beer. However, research indicates that when spirits are diluted and alcohol is added to beer to bring them to the same concentration as wine (about

12 percent), the alcohol in wine is absorbed more slowly than with either of the other two.

Alcohol does not accumulate in the blood of a non-alcoholic, healthy, well-fed person so long as consumption levels are below 8 to 10 grams per hour.

The rate of absorption is also affected by the ingestion of food. Once absorbed, about 10 percent of the alcohol is eliminated through perspiration and through breathing. The other 90 percent is metabolized by an enzyme, *alcohol dehydrogenase,* with the help of other substances from digested food. Most of this enzyme resides in the liver. However, the lining of the stomach also contains alcohol dehydrogenase, which affects the rate at which alcohol is absorbed from the stomach. Some research indicates that men have more of this enzyme than women; the result is that women will have a higher blood alcohol level than men, even when body size is taken into consideration.

Alcohol dehydrogenase is saturated when the blood alcohol level reaches 46 mg/dl (equivalent to 0.046); this amounts to about 10 grams of alcohol per hour in a 155-pound man. A woman of the same size would reach the saturation point at about two-thirds of this consumption level.

Although alcoholics metabolize alcohol faster than moderate drinkers, their livers do not produce more alcohol dehydrogenase. Research indicates that other parts of the metabolism cycle are speeded up.

However, alcohol does not accumulate in the blood of a non-alcoholic, healthy, well-fed person so long as consumption levels are below 8 to 10 grams per hour. Because alcohol dehydrogenase needs the help of substances from the digestion of food, people who have not eaten absorb alcohol faster and metabolize it more slowly. Wine is a healthier beverage because it is usually consumed with meals and because the alcohol in wine is absorbed more slowly than the alcohol in other beverages.

Harmful effects of alcohol are dose-related as are the cardio-protective effects of moderate consumption. Although it is a hypothesis at this point in medical research, many scientists feel that peak blood alcohol levels may be a major factor in determining the level where consumption crosses the line from good to bad. Some feel that the 46 mg/dl (.046 BAC) may be that line.

Certainly this is a good point to stay below. It seems to be the liver's saturation point and it's about half of the 0.08 to 0.10 maximums that most states use to determine legal intoxication for drivers.

ALCHOL CONSUMPTION AND MORTALITY

Note: The higher the number, the greater the risk

cause of death	non drinkers	occasional drinkers	1	2	3	4	5	6+	irregular drinkers
			drinks/day						
All Causes	1.00	0.88	0.84	0.93	1.02	1.08	1.22	1.38	1.01
All Cancers	1.00	0.89	0.91	1.06	1.13	1.31	1.48	1.61	1.06
Oral Cavity Cancer	1.00	1.21	0.40	1.02	2.16	3.24	2.67	6.15	1.95
Esophagus cancer	1.00	1.12	1.37	1.61	3.52	5.35	3.53	5.79	1.64
Coronary heart disease	1.00	0.86	0.79	0.80	0.83	0.74	0.85	0.92	0.96
Cerebrovascular disease	1.00	0.94	0.78	1.00	1.15	1.35	1.27	1.51	1.01
Liver cirrhosis	1.00	1.55	1.21	3.15	5.39	8.67	10.6	18.1	2.28
Suicide	1.00	1.08	1.31	1.54	1.77	2.12	2.58	2.52	1.23
Accidents	1.00	0.96	0.98	0.95	1.32	1.22	1.22	1.73	1.05

Source: BOFFETTA AND GARFINKEL, Epidemiology, September 1990

Sidebar Fourteen

Alcohol's Role in Preventing Gallstones

Gallstones are a major contributor to illness in America and the rest of the Western world. In the United States alone, more than 500,000 people endure surgery to remove these bits of calcium and cholesterol from gallbladders and bile ducts. Equally significant, numerous studies since 1979 have demonstrated that people with gallbladder disease were six to seven times more likely than other people to develop ischemic heart disease.

Numerous studies have also shown that **consumers of alcohol had dramatically less gallbladder disease, perhaps only one-third, than abstainers.** The same factors that increase the risk of heart disease also increase the risk of gallbladder disease. Indeed, both conditions occur most frequently in people with high levels of bad LDL cholesterol, triglycerides (fats) and insulin along with low levels of good HDL cholesterol.

Research has proven that moderate alcohol consumption increases HDL levels and buffers high peak insulin levels which also seem to affect gallstone disease.

TWENTY-SEVEN

Alcohol And Cancer

Does alcohol cause cancer? It depends upon whom you ask.

The International Agency for Research on Cancer (IARC), a branch of the United Nations' World Health Organization (WHO), issued a statement in 1987 that said, "the consumption of alcoholic beverages is *causally related* [emphasis in original document] to the occurrence of cancers of the oral cavity [mouth], pharynx [throat], larynx [voice box], esophagus and liver **which tend to be rare** [emphasis added]."

The IARC study found "no indication that alcohol increases the risk for cancers of the stomach, lung, urinary bladder, kidney, ovary, prostate, lymph system or blood and blood marrow." It said it found "suggestive but inconclusive" links with cancers of rectum.

A 1981 article by Doll and Petro in the *Journal of the National Cancer Institute* estimated that perhaps 3 percent of cancer deaths in the U.S. were related to alcohol. That study also estimated that another 3 percent of cancers were caused by "geophysical" factors -- such as living in Denver as opposed to Memphis. (Denver's higher altitude means that the background radiation from cosmic rays is higher than Memphis.)

But moderate consumers of alcohol don't seem to differ much from the population as a whole, except that their overall risk of dying from all causes is 10 percent lower than abstainers or heavy drinkers.

> ***A review of the evidence relied upon by the IARC working group reveals that, "the putative causal relationship between alcohol and cancer is based upon inconsistent and limited epidemiological evidence," that the animal studies fail to support a causal link and that no satisfactory explanation for a possible causal relationship has been elucidated.***

Test animals have been exposed to considerably greater amounts of alcohol than have ever been reported in epidemiological studies (the equivalent of four 25-ounce bottles of 86-proof whiskey a day for life for a 70-kg [155-pound] human) ... The animal studies have failed to support a conclusion that alcohol is carcinogenic at any level."

According to Dr. Emanuel Rubin, M.D., who is a professor and chairman of the Department of Pathology and Cell Biology at the Jefferson Medical College of Thomas Jefferson University, Philadelphia, and also Adjunct Professor of Biochemisty and Biophysics at the University of Pennsylvania Medical School:

"A review of the evidence relied upon by the IARC working group reveals that,

- "the putative causal relationship between alcohol and cancer is based upon inconsistent and limited epidemiological evidence,
- "that the animal studies fail to support a causal link and
- "that no satisfactory explanation for a possible causal relationship has been elucidated."

Dr. Rubin is not alone in his conclusions. He said that one of the biggest flaws in the IARC's conclusion is that studies of laboratory animals exposed to very high levels of alcohol consistently fail to develop cancer. Even the few that have shown a relationship have done so only at the very highest levels.

"The animal data support the hypothesis that the observed statistical associations [between alcohol and cancer] are due to the confounding factors [unconnected with alcohol] rather than the alcohol," Dr. Rubin said. "Test animals have been exposed to considerably greater amounts of alcohol than have ever been reported in epidemiological studies (the equivalent of four 25- ounce bottles of 86-proof whiskey a day for life for a 70-kg [155-pound] human) ... The animal studies have failed to support a conclusion that alcohol is carcinogenic at any level."

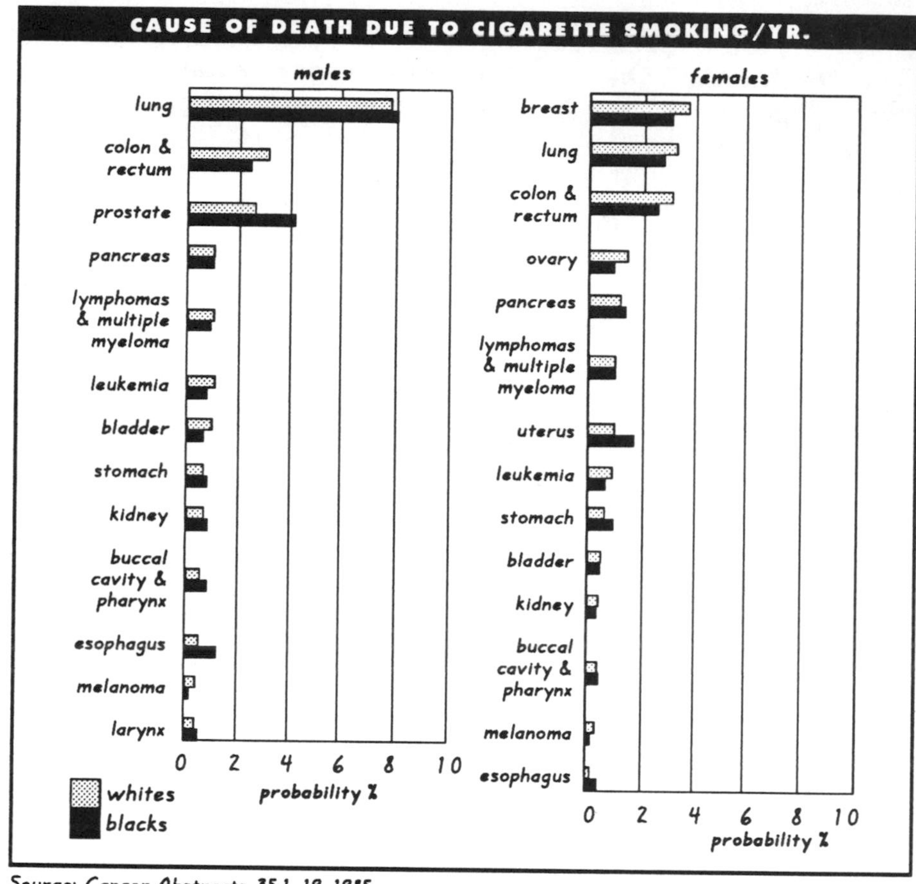

Source: *Cancer Abstracts.* 35:1. 19. 1985

As you read in this book's chapters on breast cancer and interpreting study results, epidemiological studies involve the assembly of vast amounts of data -- much of it self-reported (therefore somewhat inaccurate) -- which is analyzed using a variety of mathematical and statistical techniques. Before a scientific or public health conclusion can be based on epidemiological data, scientists use a number of other key tests to assess the credibility of the epidemiological data. Those key factors include:

- Is the conclusion verified by laboratory animal studies?
- Are the results consistent from one study to another?

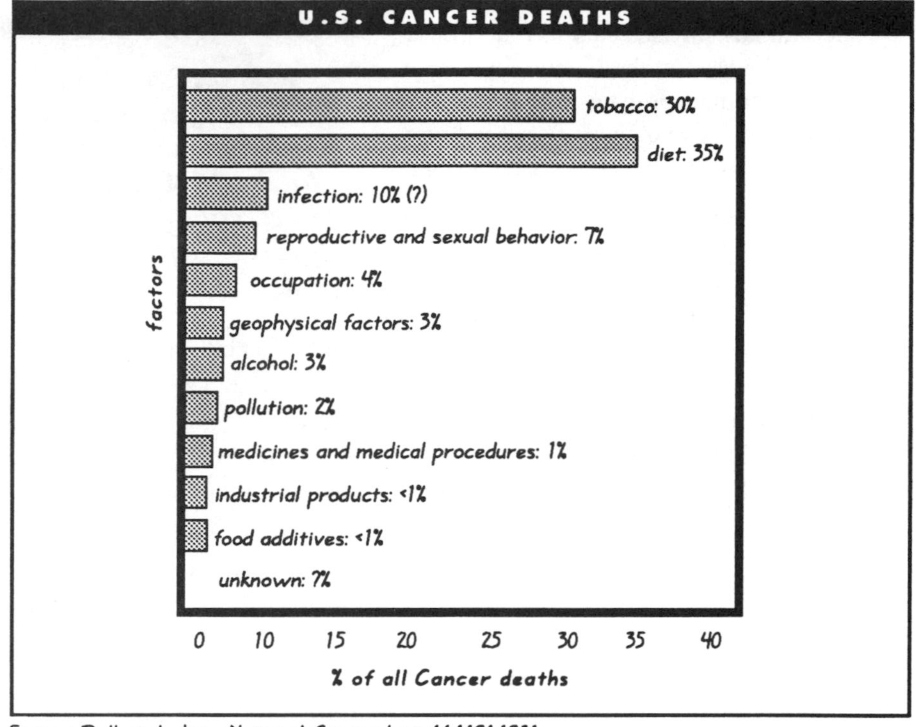

Source: Doll et.al. Jour. National Cancer Inst. 66:1191.1981

- Is the conclusion supported by the **total body** of research?
- Is the effect dose-related?
- Has the epidemiologist corrected for biases such as picking a representative sample and adjusted for confounding factors such as smoking and other related diseases?
- Is there a logical biological mechanism to explain the association?

Dr. Rubin pointed out that **animal tests repeatedly have not supported the alcohol-cancer association and that "estimates" of cancer risk in this case have not been verified.**

"At least one commentator who posits a causal link between alcohol and cancer has **estimated** [emphasis in original document] that 9 grams per kilogram of body weight per day of ethanol administered to rats would cause hepatocellular carcinomas [liver cancer] in 50 percent of the animals. In fact, rats fed alcohol at higher levels for their entire lifetimes, and subhuman primates intoxicated for more than six years have failed to show increased liver cancers," said Dr. Rubin.

It is impermissible to select from these studies only those data which support an association and ignore those that do not.

It's significant to note that 9 grams is approximately one "drink" and that a 70-kg person (155 pounds) would have to drink 70 drinks per day to reach this level -- acute alcohol poisoning and death would result before this level was reached.

The IARC studies also fail the tests of consistent results and support by the total body of research. Dr. Rubin said that the IARC was guilty of stacking the deck toward their conclusion by ignoring data that did not fit.

Dr. Rubin also points out that, although having cirrhosis of the liver puts a person at increased risk of liver cancer, "99 percent or more [of abusers] do **not** [emphasis added] get liver cancer.

"It is impermissible to select from these studies only those data which support an association and ignore those that do not. For example, the four prospective studies [used by the IARC] which report associations between the ingestion of alcoholic beverages and cancers of the oral cavity, larynx, esophagus and liver come to different conclusions."

One of these studies found an association with lung and rectal cancer and not with esophagus, stomach, colon, prostate or liver cancer. In a similar vein, other studies found an association with one type of cancer not found in other studies while finding no associations which were found in those other studies.

This lack of consistency and the failure of the total body of research to support the alcohol-cancer link may point to biases in the study, particularly the failure to control for known cancer risks.

For example, Dr. Rubin said that the primary external cause of liver cancer is the hepatitis B virus; but "**none** [emphasis added] of the studies purporting to relate the incidence of liver cancer to alcohol consumption have properly controlled for hepatitis B. Such an omission is particularly significant because there is reason to believe that the chronic alcohol abuser population has an increased prevalence of hepatitis B."

Dr. Rubin also pointed out that **heavy drinkers were almost always tobacco smokers as well and that it was impossible to get a statistically significant sample of heavy drinkers who did not also smoke**. Thus, studies that concluded that alcohol consumption was related to lung, mouth, throat and larynx cancers are probably flawed by this inability to correct.

This lack of consistency and the failure of the total body of research to support the alcohol-cancer link may point to biases in the study, particularly the failure to control for known cancer risks.

All of the other types of cancer which the IARC concludes are linked to alcohol consumption are also marred by the failure to correct for known causal links. These uncorrected-for risks include:

- mouth and oral cavity cancer risk: tobacco use, poor dental hygiene and poorly fitting dentures;
- esophageal cancer risk: nutritional deficiencies, consumption of hot (non-alcoholic) drinks, socioeconomic factors;
- colon/rectal cancer risk: diet, lack of fiber;
- breast cancer risk: causes unknown (but **not** linked to alcohol by the IARC);
- stomach cancer risk: diet, ulcers.

Finally, the studies relied upon by the IARC do not demonstrate any consistent dose relationship (except at the very highest levels of abuse) and the few mechanisms proposed as possible biological mechanisms to explain alcohol's effects have not stood up under scientific scrutiny.

Among the three most common proposed mechanisms is that alcohol is a promoter, not a prime cause, of cancer. "If it were a promoter," Dr. Rubin said, "alcohol would be expected, under these theories, to cause cell replication. In fact, alcohol does not induce cell proliferation, and, under some circumstances actually inhibits it."

A second theory proposes that ingestion of **large amounts** of alcohol (far above that of moderate consumption) causes certain enzymes, known as P-450, to act on certain non-carcinogenic molecules turning them into carcinogens. "But this theory of mechanism fails to take account of the evidence that the presence of alcohol itself inhibits the activities of the P-450 class of enzymes," said Dr. Rubin.

The few mechanisms proposed as possible biological mechanisms to explain alcohol's effects have not stood up under scientific scrutiny.

Finally, a third theory involves compounds produced by the metabolism of alcohol. The chain of chemical reactions in alcohol metabolism first produces acetaldehyde, then acetate and finally water and carbon dioxide. Acetate, carbon dioxide and water are all normal metabolites produced when the body uses most food sources. Acetaldehyde is a short-lived intermediate compound produced when alcohol is first metabolized and has an established role in metabolism. Acetaldehyde has been extensively studied and acts as a carcinogen only when **inhaled** in high concentrations.

Among other medical experts who agree with Dr. Rubin are:

♥ Dr. Parviz Pour, M.D., Professor at the University of Nebraska's Epply Institute for Research in Cancer, "... after careful analysis of the reported data in epidemiologic and laboratory studies on the possible association between alcohol and esophageal cancer, I have concluded that alcohol cannot be considered a carcinogen or co-carcinogen of the esophagus nor can it be regarded as a promoter of esophageal carcinogenesis."

♥ Dr. Michael Anderson, M.D., Senior Research Fellow, Cancer Research Campaign (the British equivalent of the American Cancer Society), who said that many of the IARC studies were "poorly designed or reported ... and that any findings in the better designed and reported studies are likely to reflect the fact that the population of chronic heavy alcohol users exposed themselves to known or unknown risk factors (poor diet, smoking, infection) not adequately accounted for in the studies."

♥ Marvin Goldman, Ph.D., Professor of Toxicology at the University of California, Davis, who said, "the overwhelming and consistent

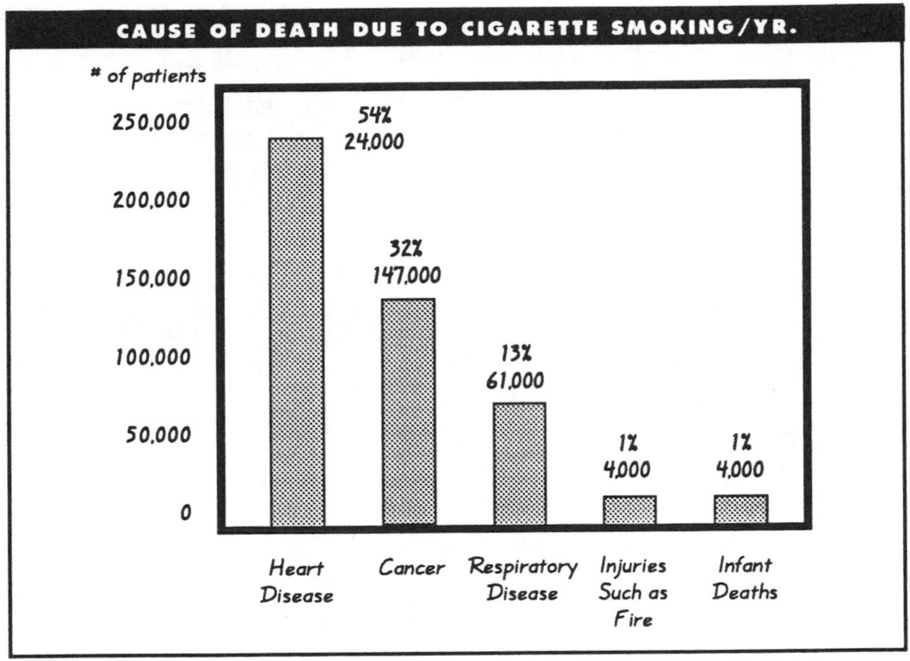

Sources: Amer. Cancer Society and U.S. DHHS

trend in the laboratory experiments is that alcohol is not a carcinogen."

♥ Paul Levy, Sc.D., Professor and Director of the Epidemiology and Biometery programs at the University of Illinois, School of Public Health, who found the IARC's conclusions were based on flawed methodology.

♥ Dr. John Doull, M.D., Ph.D., Professor and Director of the Center of Environmental and Occupational Health at the University of Kansas Medical Center who said that, the "experimental studies do not provide a basis for any conclusion other than there is, at this time, no demonstration of the carcinogenicity of alcohol."

The answer on the links between cancer and alcohol seems to be a contest of dueling scientists. Conclusions in this matter, like those in other areas, must be individual ones based on the best available information. That best information **may** indict heavy drinking, but does

not indict moderate consumption, particularly when alcohol is consumed in the absence of known cancer-causing factors such as tobacco smoking.

Making a decision is often complicated, as it is here, by scientific investigators who may have a point of view they wish to support. In this case, the World Health Organization has a publicly stated policy goal to reduce -- and if possible, eliminate -- alcohol consumption of all sorts. To link alcohol consumption with cancer would advance that organizational policy.

The IARC and other anti-alcohol activities of the WHO are also heavily funded by Islamic countries who oppose alcohol on religious grounds. On the other hand, Dr. Rubin and his colleagues have, on occasion, conducted studies that have been funded by portions of the alcoholic beverage industry.

In assessing the possible (but by no means causal) associations between the different conclusions and the possible points of view behind them, it is very important to realize that the research conducted by Dr. Rubin and his associates has been reviewed by their scientific peers (unassociated with any industry-funded research) and published in respected scientific journals. By contrast, the IARC's conclusion was not peer-reviewed, has not been published in a respected scientific journal and must be viewed as a government statement which reflects both scientific and policy considerations.

The research conducted by Dr. Rubin and his associates has been reviewed by their scientific peers (unassociated with any industry-funded research) and published in respected scientific journals. By contrast, the IARC's conclusion was not peer-reviewed, has not been published in a respected scientific journal and must be viewed as a government statement which reflects both scientific and policy considerations.

Sidebar Fifteen

Can Wine Fight Cancer?

One of nature's most potent cancer-fighting compounds, *quercetin*, has been isolated in red wine.

Research shows that quercetin, also found in onions and garlic, has the ability to block the action of the human oncogene (cancer gene) known as H-RAS and keep it from converting normal cells into cancerous ones.

According to research announced in 1991 and conducted at the University of California, Berkeley and at Georgetown University, quercetin is inactive as found in food, but is activated into its cancer-fighting form by fermentation or by bacteria in the human intestinal tract.

Epidemiological studies have liked high consumption of foods containing quercetin with lower incidences of stomach, intestine and other cancers.

"Quercetin is a powerful anti-cancer compound," said Terance Leighton, Professor of Biochemistry at the University of California, Berkeley, who led the study. "There is even some suggestion that compounds, such as quercetin and others, may be responsible for the reduced levels of coronary artery disease found among moderate wine consumers."

In a study conducted by researchers at Cornell University, the potential for wine to prevent cancer was demonstrated in laboratory mice. The investigators were studying the ability of ethyl carbamate (also known as urethane) to cause cancer. Since ethyl carbamate is present in trace amounts in some wines, they administered this substance to the animals in several ways: in water, in plain alcohol, in white wine and in red wine. The animals receiving the ethyl carbonate in water and in alcohol had higher levels of cancer than the control animals. Those receiving it in white wine actually had **lower** levels of cancer than the controls. Those receiving it in red wine had the lowest levels of all!

TWENTY-EIGHT

Wine and Lead

The issue of lead in wine became front-page news in 1991 in most American newspapers, despite the fact that most wine contains lower concentrations than scores of other common foods including homemade spaghetti sauce, oranges, spinach or whole wheat bread.

The controversy started when a San Diego law firm forced the U.S. Bureau of Alcohol, Tobacco and Firearms (BATF), which regulates all alcoholic beverages, to release preliminary test data on lead concentrations in wine.

The publicity over lead in wine is comparable to the scare over Alar on apples which was later shown to have been a tempest in a teapot.

The BATF did so reluctantly, asserting that their tests had not been conducted in a scientifically valid manner and that the results were inaccurate and probably unreliable.

But unreliable as the data were, the public firestorm that followed resulted in press conferences by the Food and Drug Administration (FDA) and the eventual establishment of an interim standard for lead in wine of 300 parts per billion (ppb). By the time you read this, a permanent standard of 150 ppb will probably have been established.

What effect will all this have? Little to none, at least for American wines which, in the BATF tests, showed an average of 41 ppb (with California wines about half of that). Imported wines had higher lead levels, averaging about 94 ppb.

The levels of lead were higher for wine poured from bottles with a lead-foil capsule sealing the neck. Those capsules, however, are on their way out and will not be seen on most wine bottled after Dec. 31, 1992.

The FDA's activities on wine and lead are "Mickey Mouse," according to Dr. Curtis Klaassen, professor of pharmacology and toxicology at the University of Kansas Medical School.

Older wines which still have lead capsules are safe, but you should wipe down the bottle mouth with a paper or cloth rag before pouring the wine

Experts Say Lead In Wine Poses No Danger

Most medical and scientific experts say the publicity over lead in wine is comparable to the scare over Alar on apples which was later shown to have been a tempest in a teapot.

The FDA's activities on wine and lead are "Mickey Mouse," according to Dr. Curtis Klaassen, professor of pharmacology and toxicology at the University of Kansas Medical School. Dr. Klaassen is also the author of the section dealing with lead and heavy metals in the respected medical reference book, *The Pharmacological Basis of Therapeutics*, used and consulted by most American physicians (published by MacMillan Publishing, Goodman and Gilman, editors).

"Environmental lead is an issue for children, not adults," said Dr. Klaassen who added that **lead levels in wine were "irrelevant from a health standpoint."**

Dr. Klaassen said the FDA emphasis should be on protecting children, who are far more susceptible to lead than adults. He also pointed out that lead deposited in the bones of a woman before she becomes pregnant could be dissolved and transferred to the fetus during pregnancy, but only if she eats a diet deficient in calcium. "With the proper amount of calcium, the lead stays in place."

"It's [FDA lead/wine actions] a high-profile issue that gets them headlines and makes some points with the anti-alcohol groups," said a professor of medicine at Yale University Medical School who wished to remain anonymous to avoid jeopardizing government research grants. "In my opinion they're wasting a lot of time, money and effort that could be better spent on a real problem -- protecting our kids."

Other medical experts have previously expressed their doubts about the relevance of lead in wine.

"If you drink enough wine for lead to be a problem, you've got a hell of an alcohol abuse problem," said Dr. John Osterloh, Associate Professor at the University of California, San Francisco Medical School.

"If you drink enough wine for lead to be a problem, you've got a hell of an alcohol abuse problem," — Dr. John Osterloh, Associate Professor at the University of California, San Francisco Medical School

FDA Is Guessing, Basing Its Conclusion About Lead in Wine On Incorrect, Incomplete, Outdated and Nonexistent Data

The FDA's standard for lead in wine -- indeed all their standards governing low levels of lead -- are part guesswork, part science, and partly based on old, conflicting or incorrect data. The standards may or may not have a medically defensible relationship to the health effects of lead in concentrations found in water, wine or other foods.

But these standards are probably the best the government can come up with, given the faulty state of information and scientific research, said the more than 40 state and federal government officials and medical school experts we interviewed.

As a microcosm of government standards-setting, an investigation of the interim lead/wine standard casts serious doubts on the reliability of the data used to establish safety and tolerance levels and raises serious questions about whether the public is adequately served.

What's Safe? No One Knows

"There is no definite answer on how much lead can be safely consumed," said Dr. Dan Paschal at the Atlanta-based Centers For Disease Control (CDC). "The research is not conclusive. We don't know what to measure."

Different federal government agencies do not agree on the basic data on which the standards- setting process is based.

"What's safe?" asked Dr. Osterloh. "The bottom line is that there are no definitive studies and possibly no way to do studies on the effects of lead as low as they are in wine. What's safe? I don't think anybody knows."

"No one really knows what level is healthy," said Rich Nickle of the Agency for Toxic Substances and Disease Registry (ATSDR), a part of the U.S. Public Health Service (PHS).

The FDA had no comment on the soundness of their standard levels or on the validity of the data on which the standards are based.

Numerous telephone calls to the FDA to discuss this situation were not returned.

Government Agencies Disagree

In addition, our interviews found that different federal government agencies do not agree on the basic data on which the standards- setting process is based. Specifically, different government agencies cited different numbers for:

- the average amount of lead ingested by the U.S. population in general,
- the average level of lead in the bloodstream and
- the blood concentration levels at which health effects from lead start to evidence themselves.

The only generally agreed-upon number defined the relationship between the amount of lead ingested and the corresponding increase in adult blood lead levels. According to the "Uptake Biokinetic Model" developed by the EPA, if an average 150 pound adult consumes one microgram (millionth of a gram) of lead, the blood lead level will increase by 0.32 micrograms-per-liter.

According to the EPA's Jeff Cohen who helped develop the information, the Uptake Biokinetic Model takes absorption of lead and excretion into account.

The U.S. Center for Health Statistics, a part of the PHS, said they "had no idea of what the levels might be" and didn't know where to look.

Research and medical professions generally measure blood lead levels in micrograms-per-**deci**liter, one-tenth of a liter. But since micrograms-per-liter is equivalent to parts-per-billion (ppb), and since ppb is the most common unit of concentration used for measurements in food by the FDA, water by the EPA and lead measurements by the BATF, this chapter will use micrograms- per-liter for blood lead levels for consistency and to help avoid confusion.

Investigation Yields Conflicting Numbers

The significance of the EPA's Uptake Biokinetic Model is hard to determine when agencies can't agree on what is a safe level in the blood, how much lead people consume or even what is the average blood level.

The U.S. Center for Health Statistics, a part of the PHS, said they "had no idea of what the levels might be" and didn't know where to look.

ATSDR's Nickle, however, said that numbers for their 1988 "Toxicological Profile of Lead" indicated that blood lead levels might be as high as 170 to 200 micrograms-per-liter, but that other research indicated it might be as low as 60 to 80 micrograms-per-liter.

The ATSDR research indicated that people in remote societies, such as one studied in the Himalayas, had blood lead levels as low as 34 micrograms-per-liter. In their "1988 Report to Congress" that same study indicated that, in general, people in industrialized nations had blood lead levels from 100 to 170 micrograms-per-liter.

Estimates of the average daily intake of lead also vary wildly. According to Ellis Gunderson of the FDA's Contaminate Chemistry Division, the average American consumes about 7 micrograms of lead daily with the figure closer to 6 for women and 8 for men. But that number is not universally accepted.

"I find that hard to believe," said UCSF's Dr. Osterloh, who was the most vocal of more than a dozen skeptics. Many of the other skeptics were officials in federal and state government agencies who seemed reluctant to publicly criticize the FDA. "The average person would get more than that by drinking a quart of water," said Dr. Osterloh. "I'd think the figure was closer to 50."

The significance of the EPA's Uptake Biokinetic Model is hard to determine when agencies can't agree on what is a safe level in the blood, how much lead people consume or even what is the average blood level.

Other government statistics seem to back up Dr. Osterloh. According to the ATSDR, an EPA study published in 1988 indicated that the average adult male consumed 50.7 micrograms of lead per day and the average female, 37.5, the difference accounted for by the amount of food eaten.

Scenario Conflicts With FDA Estimate

While overall lead intake has dropped in the United States due to the phasing out of leaded gasoline and the declining use of lead-soldered food cans, Dr. Osterloh's suspicions seem justified when examined in light of other government figures.

For example, the current EPA standard for drinking water is 50 ppb. The EPA has also established a new "action level" of 15 ppb to go into effect in 1992.

If a person drank a liter of water per day (a liter is 1.06 quarts) containing 7.5 ppb of lead (half of the EPA action level) then they would consume 7.5 micrograms of lead in the water alone. Since EPA standards are based on the assumption that a person drinks two quarts per day, this scenario would have that person consuming 15 micrograms per day just from water alone, a figure that is twice the FDA's estimates.

In addition, the 7.5 ppb assumption for lead concentrations in water may be toward the low end of reality. According to the ATSDR's 1990 "Toxicological Profile For Lead" prepared in collaboration with the EPA, the average U.S. public water system contains 5 ppb at the source with tap water concentration in homes and schools averaging from 10 to 30 ppb.

Spinach, for example, contains 39 ppb of lead; a person consuming four ounces would add 4.2 micrograms of lead. A two-ounce white bread roll, measured by the FDA at 28 ppb, would add another 3 micrograms.

Finally, using the FDA's numbers for some common foods quickly raises the average person's intake. Spinach, for example, contains 39 ppb of lead; a person consuming four ounces would add 4.2 micrograms of lead. A two-ounce white bread roll, measured by the FDA at 28 ppb, would add another 3 micrograms. Using these figures, it is easy to see why Dr. Osterloh and others doubt the FDA numbers for total daily intake.

EPA Model Seems To Contradict FDA

If the EPA's Uptake Biokinetic Model is valid, then it should be possible to work backwards to determine what level of lead intake is necessary to raise blood lead to a given level. If we take a conservative blood lead level, 60 micrograms-per-liter, and divide it by 0.32 (from the Uptake Biokinetic Model's formula), then a person would have to consume 187.5 micrograms-per-day to maintain this blood lead level, which many estimates indicate may be too low for the United States.

"It Doesn't Compute"

Clearly either the FDA consumption data is incorrect, the EPA model is not valid or the ATSDR's blood level data is incorrect.

"It doesn't compute, does it?" commented a source within the FDA who requested that his name not be used. "Now you know why it took us so long to come up with a number (for the lead/wine standard). It's very confusing and we don't have all the facts we need to make the

"It's very confusing and we don't have all the facts we need to make the decision," said the source, who was part of the team which developed the interim lead standard for wine.

decision," said the source, who was part of the team which developed the interim lead standard for wine.

While all health experts agreed that lead plays no useful role in the human body and that the less lead consumed the better, opinions vary widely about what is safe, what is tolerable and what levels should be set by regulatory bodies.

Acute lead poisoning is fairly easy to diagnose and regulate. According to the ATSDR's "Toxicological Profile For Lead," blood lead levels of more than 400 micrograms-per-liter cause anemia, neurological disturbances, kidney and reproductive damage.

This 400 micrograms-per-liter level is recognized as the maximum acceptable occupational level by the federal Occupational Safety and Health Administration (OSHA).

"You need to realize that this level is not necessarily a 'safe' level," said Dr. Michael Montopoli of the National Institute of Occupational Safety and Health. "Occupational standards must balance medical considerations with the economic impact on industry and the feasibility of current technology to deal with it. However, there is some debate as to whether the current standard should be lowered."

The ATSDR's "Toxicological Profile For Lead" shows health effects dropping off rapidly below 250 micrograms-per-liter. However, at this level the study indicates that the lead could still cause high blood pressure.

"The EPA bandies about a number of 10 micrograms-per-deciliter (100 micrograms-per-liter) as a defacto acceptable number," said CDC's Dr. Paschal. "But that's a number of convenience. There may be no threshold (safe level) for lead."

According to *Neurotoxicology,* a reference book by EPA Senior Scientist J.M. Davis, 100 micrograms-per-liter represents a level of low observed effects, but then goes on to state that there may not exist a level with **no** observed effects. In other words, lead may not have a safety threshold.

According to the "Toxicological Profile for Lead" the only known medical effect for blood lead concentrations less than 100 micrograms-per-liter may the inhibition of ALA-D, an enzyme involved in the production of red blood cells. "There may be an actual health effect or there may not be," said ATSDR's Nickle.

Medical reference books indicate that inhibition of ALA-D may be connected to high blood pressure which, in turn, has a well-known connection to cardiovascular disease. However, as you have already read in this book, the overwhelming body of research has proved that moderate drinkers have lower cardiovascular death rates than abstainers and heavy drinkers. Indeed, increased blood pressures are only seen in heavy drinkers.

In everyday terms, linear regression analysis works like this: research indicates that if 100,000 people fell off a 1,000-foot cliff, they would all die. If they fell off a 500-foot cliff, 50,000 would die. If they fell from a 100-foot cliff, 10,000 would die. If taken to its lowest levels, then 100 people would die if the cliff was only one foot high and 10 people would die if it were only one-tenth of a foot.

The method, scientists point out, works in some cases but not in all cases (such as the cliff example).

Linear Regressive Analysis May Or May Not Be Valid

Dr. Osterloh and several other government scientists said they didn't have a lot of faith in "the curve" at lower blood lead concentrations -- especially below 100 micrograms-per-liter. Part of this, they explained, was the reliance on what's known as linear regressive analysis in which the results at high concentrations are

Scientists have increasingly found that in some cases mechanisms come into play that can effectively neutralize a chemical at low concentrations which is poisonous at higher levels.

extrapolated backwards to lower concentrations -- perhaps concentrations that are too low to measure directly with current technology.

However, as technology advances, scientists have increasingly found that in some cases mechanisms come into play that can effectively neutralize a chemical at low concentrations which is poisonous at higher levels.

This linear regressive analysis is frequently used with substances like lead or low-level radiation which are thought to have no safety threshold.

In everyday terms, linear regression analysis works like this: research indicates that if 100,000 people fell off a 1,000-foot cliff, they would all die. If they fell off a 500-foot cliff, 50,000 would die. If they fell from a 100-foot cliff, 10,000 would die. If taken to its lowest levels, then 100 people would die if the cliff was only one foot high and 10 people would die if it were only one-tenth of a foot.

The method, scientists point out, works in some cases but not in all cases (such as the cliff example).

So How Safe Is Wine?

The proven fact that moderate consumers of alcohol have a 10 percent or more reduced risk of dying **from all causes** and that wine drinkers have the same -- or perhaps better -- odds indicates that lead in wine has **no effect** at all. Moreover, even alcoholics have not been found to suffer from lead-related problems. A European study found that alcoholics who drank mostly wine had higher, but non-toxic, blood lead levels than other alcoholics.

But like all scientific problems, answering this question requires a certain set of assumptions. Obviously, the results are wrong if the assumptions are incorrect. And as we have seen, the government's numbers don't always compute.

But for the sake of this argument, assume that:

- A bottle of wine contains 21 ppb lead (the California average).
- 21 ppb is equivalent to 21 micrograms-per-liter, which equals 15.75 micrograms in a 750-ml bottle.
- A 750-ml bottle contains six drinks of wine.
- One glass of wine contains 2.63 micrograms of lead.

The proven fact that moderate consumers of alcohol have a 10 percent or more reduced risk of dying* from all causes *and that wine drinkers have the same -- or perhaps better -- odds indicates that lead in wine has* no effect *at all.

If the EPA's Uptake Biokinetic Model is correct, a person drinking a glass of this wine every day could expect an increase in the blood lead level of 2.63 X 0.32 or 0.84 micrograms-per- liter. This compares to an average blood lead level which may be between 60 and 170 micrograms-per-liter. The 0.84 increase may be considered **not** significant in relation to the overall blood lead level.

Time and again, experts said, "there are no definitive studies," and "We need better science before we can find solid answers."

Until then, wine -- alone among all foods and beverages which contain equal or greater amounts of lead -- remains singled out for the sort of government attention which most experts say is a waste of time.

PART IV
Cooking With The French Paradox

Dilled Asparagus

Serves 4

1 lb. asparagus
1 pat butter, sliced thinly
1/4 t. dill
Salt and pepper to taste

Put cleaned asparagus in a glass loaf pan. Place butter slices on top. Sprinkle with dill, salt and pepper. Cover and microwave at 50 percent for 3 minutes. Toss lightly. Microwave for another 3 minutes. Let stand for 4-5 minutes before serving.

Asparagus Rice Soup

Serves 4

1 lb. asparagus
1 1/2 c. basamati rice
1 T. olive oil
1 small yellow onion
1 t. minced garlic
1 t. parsley or chervil
9 cups water
1/2 c. shredded Parmesan cheese.

Wash and chop asparagus into one inch pieces reserving the top 3 inches. Saute onion, garlic and parsley until onion is slightly browned. Add water and the bottom pieces of the asparagus. Bring to a boil and cook for 15 minutes. Add basamati rice. Bring to a boil. Simmer for at least 20 minutes covered. When rice is cooked bring back to a boil and add asparagus tips. Cook for 3 minutes. Top with shredded Parmesan cheese and serve.

Black Bean Stew

Serves 4 to 6

1 large yellow onion, coarsely chopped
1 t. minced garlic
1 T. olive oil
1 yellow bell pepper
2 15-oz. cans black beans
1 t. oregano
2 t. ground cumin
1/4 t. ground coriander
1 c. carrots, sliced 1/4 inch thick (fresh or frozen)
Salt and pepper to taste

Saute onions, garlic and olive oil in a pot until onions are slightly browned. Core, seed and chop bell pepper into 1 inch thick chunks. Add to browned onions. Saute for one minute at medium high heat. Add black beans, spices and carrots. Cover and bring to a simmer. Simmer for 30 minutes. Serve hot.

Broccoli Italiano

Serves 4

1 lb. broccoli
1 T olive oil
2 1/2 t. dried basil
1/4 c. pine nuts
1/4 c. grated Parmesan cheese
Salt and pepper to taste

Cut broccoli stems in small chunks or slices and make tops into florettes. Place in a glass bowl and cover. Microwave until bright green, approximately 4 to 7 minutes. Mix basil, pine nuts and cheese together. Put mixture in a hot skillet with the broccoli and stir fry in oil until pinenuts start to brown. Salt and pepper to taste. Serve hot.

Avocado Bruchetta

Serves 4

8 1/4 inch slices of bread from a baguette (sweet or sourdough)
Garlic olive oil (see recipe in this book)
1 ripe avocado
1 T. lemon juice
2 green onions, tops trimmed, finely cut
1/4 t. red pepper flakes, crushed
Salt to taste

Brush bread lightly with garlic olive oil and toast.

Peel avocado. Mash in a bowl with chopped green onion, lemon juice and salt. Spread on toast and drizzle with a few drops of olive oil over top.

Garbanzo Chard Soup

Serves 4

2 T. olive oil
1 medium yellow onion, diced
1 t. garlic, chopped
1 10-oz. package chopped chard
2 4-oz. cans mushrooms
1 15-oz. can garbanzo beans
1 14-oz. can whole peeled tomatoes (Italian plumb preferred) cut into chunks
5 cups water
Salt and pepper to taste
Grated Parmesan cheese for garnish

Saute olive oil, onion and garlic in a soup pot. Cook over medium heat until onions are golden. Microwave chard for 5 minutes in a glass bowl covered with plastic wrap. Set aside. Add mushrooms to pot and saute for 2 minutes. Add chard, stir and cook for 2 to 3 minutes. Add garbanzo beans and tomatoes (including the juice from the can) and increase heat to high.

Add water. Bring to boil and simmer for 40 minutes with lid partly on. Add salt and pepper to taste. Serve with grated Parmesan cheese on top.

Chicken Curry

Serves 4

4 cloves garlic, crushed
1 T. olive oil
1 yellow onion (medium size)
1 can white meat chicken
2 packages dry chicken broth
2 c. water
1 T. curry powder
1/2 t. ground ginger
1/4 t. tumeric
1/4 t. crushed red pepper
1 c. basamati rice (rinsed)
2 c. green peas (frozen)
1 c. sliced carrots (frozen)
1/2 red pepper (cubed)
1/2 green pepper (cubed)

Saute garlic, oil and onion and a large pot. Add chicken and saute until onion is transparent. Add water and chicken broth packages. Bring to a boil. Add spices and rice. Bring to a second boil. Cook until rice is done. Add vegetables and cook until vegetables are cooked through.

Fennel with Cheese

Serves 4

2 large unblemished fennel bulbs with stems (about 1 lb. each)
1/4 c. olive oil
Salt and pepper to taste
1/4 cup Parmesan cheese

Trim stems from fennel then cut lengthwise into quarter wedges. Arrange wedges on a baking pan. Brush with oil and then sprinkle with salt and pepper.

Place under broiler about 8 inches from the heat until tender. Sprinkle with cheese and return to the broiler until cheese has melted.

Minestrone Soup

Serves 12

1 large yellow onion, coarsely chopped
1 T. diced garlic
2 T. olive oil
2 large zucchini, diced
1 10-oz. package Swiss chard
1 10-oz. package carrots, sliced
1 10-oz. small pasta (shells or fussili are especially good)
1 28-oz. can Italian plum tomatoes, diced
1 19-oz. can fava beans (may use kidney or canelli beans)
1 15-oz. can garbanzo beans
1/2 t. dried basil
1/2 T. dried oregano
1 t. crushed red pepper
1/2 t. dried parsley
2 packages dried beef broth
30 cups water
Salt and pepper to taste
1 10-oz. package broccoli florettes
1 10-oz. package brussel sprouts or cabbage
Grated Parmesan cheese

Saute onion, garlic and oil in a large pot. Add diced zucchini and saute until done. Add water, carrots, chard, pasta, tomatoes, beans, garbanzos and spices. Cook about one hour or until all ingredients are cooked through. Add broccoli and brussel sprouts. Cook for another 10 minutes. Serve hot topped with grated Parmesan cheese.

Oven Broiled Mushrooms with Garlic, Oregano and Parmesan

Serves 4

1 lb. mushrooms, fresh, whole
1 t. olive oil
2 t. minced garlic
1 T. olive oil
1/2 t. dried oregano
1/2 c. grated Parmesan cheese

Wash mushrooms and cut off stems. Place on a foil-covered lightly oiled cookie sheet, close together with the stem side up. Mix garlic and olive oil in a small bowl. Brush mushrooms with mixture (you can put the leftovers in a jar to use at another time). Crush oregano and mix with cheese. Sprinkle cheese mixture evenly over mushrooms mounding on top of caps. Place under broiler about six inches below the broiler unit until cheese is melted and slightly brown and mushrooms are warmed through (approximately 6 minutes).

Grilled Salmon with Artichoke Hearts

Serves 2

1/2 lb. salmon fillet
Juice of 1/2 lemon
2 T. olive oil
1 t. minced garlic
1/4 t. dried marjoram
1/4 t. thyme
1/4 t. red pepper flakes
1/4 t. salt
1/4 t. cracked black pepper
1/4 c. white wine
1/2 of a 6.5-oz. jar of artichoke hearts marinated in oil and vinegar with leaves removed and hearts cut into 1/4 to 1/2 inch pieces

Mix salt, pepper and spices with 1 T. olive oil and the lemon juice. Spread over salmon and marinate for 15 minutes. Scrape off marinade and save. Cook salmon in a pan at very high heat with the skin side down for 3 minutes.

Turn fillet and cook for another 3 minutes. Remove skin from fillet. Turn salmon again and cook for another 3 minutes or until cooked through. Remove salmon from skillet and place on warming plate in oven.

Wipe skillet clean, then add marinade, wine and artichoke hearts. Reduce to a sauce. Pour over salmon and serve.

NOTE: The portions of the artichoke hearts which are removed for this recipe can be eaten along with the rest of the jar of artichokes as part of an antipasto platter before the meal.

Tomato and Mozzarella Plate

Serves 4

4 Italian plum tomatoes, a handful of cherry tomatoes or one beef tomato, sliced
4 oz. fresh mozzarella, sliced
Garlic olive oil (see recipe in this book)
Balsamic vinegar (or red wine vinegar)
Dried basil
Salt and pepper to taste
1/4 c. red onion, sliced
8 Kalamata olives

Place tomatoes on a plate. Put mozzarella slices on top. Drizzle with garlic olive oil and balsamic vinegar. Sprinkle lightly with basil, salt and pepper. Garnish with red onion and olives.

NOTE: You can use the Balsamic Vinegar Salad Dressing in this book instead of the garlic olive oil and spices listed above for a slightly different flavor.

Grilled Tuna with Olives

Serves 4

4 tuna steaks (about 6 oz. each) 1-inch thick
3 T. olive oil
1/2 t. dry thyme
1/2 t. dry rosemary
1 T. minced garlic
2 T. finely chopped green onion or red onion
1 T. finely chopped Kalamata olives
1 T. finely chopped capers
1/2 t. finely chopped anchovy fillets or anchovy paste
2 T. balsamic vinegar
2.t. dried parsley
1/2 c. white wine

Mix ingredients reserving 1 tablespoon of olive oil and the white wine. Cover tuna with mixture and cover with plastic wrap for at least 15 minutes. After marinating, scrape off marinade mixture and reserve.

Put 1 tablespoon olive oil in a skillet and heat. Place tuna in skillet and cook about 3 minutes. Turn and cook for another 3 minutes. When steaks are cooked through, place on a warm plate in the oven. Add reserved marinade and wine to skillet and reduce to the consistency of salsa. Pour over tuna and serve.

Zinfandel Chicken

Serves 4

2 T. flour
Salt and pepper to taste
4 skinless, boneless chicken breasts
2 T. olive oil
2 4 oz. cans mushrooms or 8 oz. fresh mushrooms, sliced
6 garlic cloves, peeled and minced
2 T. balsamic vinegar
3/4 c. chicken broth
1 bay leaf
1/4 t. dry thyme
1 c. zinfandel wine (or other red wine)
Salt and pepper to taste

Season flour with salt and pepper. Roll chicken in flour mixture shaking off excess. Heat olive oil in a skillet over medium high heat and cook chicken breasts until browned, approximately 2 to 3 minutes on each side. Add mushrooms and garlic to skillet. Cook until mushrooms are softened stirring to keep from burning (about 3 minutes). Remove chicken and place on a warming plate in the oven. Add balsamic vinegar, wine, broth, bay leaf and thyme to skillet. Cook over a medium heat until liquid reduces to a sauce. Place chicken on a plate. Pour mushroom sauce over top after discarding the bay leaf.

Asparagus with Tarragon Butter

Serves 4

1 lb. asparagus
1 T. butter
1/2 t. dried tarragon
Salt and pepper to taste

Snap off tough ends of asparagus. Place in a glass 9in x 9in glass baking dish. Sprinkle with tarragon, dot with butter. Cover and microwave for 4 to 4 1/2 minutes stirring at 2 minutes. Add salt and pepper to taste. Serve with butter left in dish poured over asparagus.

Garlic Asparagus

Serves 4

1 T. olive oil
6 cloves (approx. 1 T.) minced garlicd
1 lb. asparagus
1/2 c. water

Heat pan then add oil. When oil is hot, add garlic. Saute briefly then add asparagus. Saute quickly until asparagus is covered with oil. Add water, cover and steam for about 3 minutes or until asparagus is done. Place asparagus on a dish and pour garlic sauce over asparagus.

NOTE: This recipe is also good with broccoli.

Balsamic Vinegar Salad Dressing

1 clove garlic
1 shallot
1 t. salt
1 t. sugar
1/2 t. finely ground pepper
1/4 c. balsamic vinegar
1/4 c. seasoned or plain rice wine vinegar
1/2 c. extra virgin olive oil
1/2 c. canola oil

For a chunky dressing, mince garlic and shallot in food processor or blender, then mix with the remaining ingredients in a small bowl with a wire whip. For a smooth dressing, process all ingredients in a food processor or blender. If using a seasoned rice wine vinegar or a very sweet balsamic vinegar you can omit the sugar.

NOTE: This also makes a great marinade and baste for grilled meats.

Broccoflower

Serves 4

1 head broccoflower
1 1/2 T. olive oil
6 cloves (approx. 1 T.) minced garlic
1/2 red bell pepper (green or yellow if red not available) cored, seeded and coarsely chopped
1/2 t. crushed red pepper flakes
1 small yellow onion, diced
1/4 c. pine nuts

Break broccoflower into small florets and microwave for approximately 3 1/2 minutes or until done. Saute red pepper flakes and pine nuts in olive oil until nuts are browned. Add onion, bell pepper and garlic. Saute until onion is translucent. Add broccoflower. Stir until coated with mixture.

NOTE: Cauliflower or broccoli may be used if broccoflower is not available. If you don't have a microwave you can use the following:

Saute vegetables as directed above. Then add broccoflower. Saute for a moment, then add 1/2 cup water, cover and steam for 4 to 5 minutes, or until done.

Chicken Cacciatore

Serves 4

1 chicken, cut into eight pieces, or 2 1/2 lbs. boneless, skinless chicken pieces plus 2 T. olive oil
Salt and pepper to taste
1 c. red wine
3 to 4 c. spaghetti sauce (from this book)

In a very hot non-stick pan, brown chicken pieces for about 5 minutes. If using the boneless, skinless chicken pieces, saute in very hot olive oil until golden.

Turn over and cook until chicken is nicely browned on both sides. Drain off excess oil or fat. Salt and pepper to taste and add wine. Bring to a simmer, reduce heat and cook until done but still juicy, about 25 minutes. Heat spaghetti sauce. Place chicken on a platter and pour heated spaghetti sauce over chicken.

NOTE: When cooking skinless chicken it is imperative to brown the chicken well in very hot olive oil. Otherwise, the chicken just steams in its own juice and will turn out dry and flavorless.

Chicken in Red Wine Sauce

Serves 4

1 T. olive oil
1 yellow onion, coarsely chopped
1 t. minced garlic
1 lb. chicken breasts, boned and skinned
1 8-oz. can mushrooms (or 1 c. fresh mushrooms cut into quarters)
1 6-oz. can ripe tomatoes, cut into 1/2 inch pieces
1/4 t. thyme
1/4 t. tarragon
1/4 t. rosemary
1/4 t. parsley
1/2 c. red wine
1/4 c. black Mediterranean olives
Salt and pepper to taste
Arrowroot for thickening

Saute garlic and onions in olive oil at medium high heat until garlic starts to brown. Add chicken and cook for 3 minutes on each side until brown. Remove chicken to a heated plate. Add mushrooms to skillet and brown. Add tomatoes, wine and spices and olives. Simmer covered for 5 minutes. Remove from heat and thicken with arrowroot. Serve sauce over chicken or on the side.

Spicy Shallot Couscous

Serves 4

1/2 yellow onion, coarsely chopped
4 cloves garlic, minced
1/2 red or green bell pepper, finely chopped
1/2 c. chopped shallots or green onions (approx. 2 onions with tops)
1 T. olive oil
1 c. couscous
1 1/4 c. water
1 package chicken broth
1/2 t. red pepper flakes

Saute onion, garlic, pepper and shallots in olive oil until onions are wilted. Add couscous, water, broth and red pepper flakes. Bring to a boil, stir and cover. Remove from heat and allow to sit for 5 minutes or until water is absorbed. Fluff couscous and serve.

NOTE: You can use low salt/low fat canned chicken broth instead of the water and chicken broth package if canned is available.

Dipping Oil for Bread

3 T. extra virgin olive oil
2 T. balsamic vinegar
2 cloves garlic, crushed fresh
1/2 t. red pepper flakes
1 t. mixed dried Italian spices (oregano, thyme, rosemary, sage, basil)

Mix all ingredients together. Place in a shallow dish for dipping bread. This will keep in the refrigerator for a long time. Can also be used to toast old bread into terrific toast or croutons.

NOTE: This can also be used as a base for a marinade or a pasta glaze.

Green Beans Provencal

Serves 4

1 lb. green beans
1 lb. tomatoes
1 T. olive oil
1 T. minced garlic
1 bay leaf
Salt and pepper to taste

Cut beans into 2 inch lengths. Microwave covered on high for 4 minutes or until cooked but still crispy. Cut tomatoes into 1/2 inch cubes. Saute garlic in olive oil until garlic is lightly browned. Add tomatoes, bay leaf salt and pepper. Cook about 3 to 4 minutes. Add beans. Stir to mix. Serve warm.

Italian Beans

Serves 6

1 lb. green beans, cut into 2 inch lengths
1/4 t. powdered oregano, or
1 1/2 t. fresh
1 1/2 T. olive oil
2 t. minced garlic

Microwave beans on high for 5 minutes. On high heat saute garlic in olive oil until garlic is slightly browned. Add beans and oregano. Saute for 2 minutes. Add salt and pepper to taste.

NOTE: You can dress up this recipe by adding 1/2 cup chopped, seeded fresh tomato before the last 2 minutes of the saute. Leftovers can be reheated or served cold with a sprinkle of lemon juice or wine vinegar. Leftovers are also excellent in the Couscous Nicoise recipe in this book.

Rosemary Lamb Chops

Serves 2

1 T. olive oil
6 cloves (approx. 1 T.) minced garlic
1 t. dried rosemary
4 lamb loin chops (approx. 1 pound)
Salt and pepper to taste
1/4 c. balsamic vinegar
2 T. red wine

Saute garlic and rosemary in olive oil until garlic is toasted. Add lamb chops and grill 4 minutes, turn, add salt and pepper to grilled side and continue to grill for another 4 to 5 minutes. Put lamb chops on a warm plate in oven. Deglaze pan by adding vinegar and wine, reduce at high heat until liquid makes a sauce. Pour over lamb chops and serve.

Garlic Lentil Soup with Cloves and Bay

Serves 8 to 10

3 c. yellow onion, coarsely chopped
1 T. minced garlic
2 T. olive oil
2 c. dried lentils
3 c. tomato juice
4 c. water
1 t. salt
1/2 t. coarse black pepper
1 bay leaf
1 clove, crushed (about 1/16t)
1/2 t. dried oregano
1/4 t. celery seed
1 T. lemon juice
1 c. plain yogurt
1/4 c. chopped parsley

Rinse and drain lentils. Saute onion and garlic in oil over medium high heat until soft (about 5 minutes). Add tomato juice, water and lentils. Bring to a boil and add salt, pepper, bay leaf, clove, oregano and celery seed. Reduce heat to medium. Cover and simmer approximately 45 minutes until lentils are tender. Soup will be thick. Add another cup of water if needed.

Stir in lemon juice. Serve in heated soup bowls and garnish with a dollop of plain yogurt and chopped fresh parsley.

Coucous Nicoise

Serves 6

(Excellent leftovers for lunch)

3 c. cooked couscous (could be leftovers from another recipe in this book)
2 c. cool green beans, sliced into 1 inch sections
1/2 c. Kalamata (or other Mediterranean black olives) chopped into quarters
2 c. cherry tomatoes cut into halves
1 6 1/2 oz. jar marinated artichoke hearts, drained and cut into quarters
1 6 oz. can water packed light tuna, drained
1 medium red onion chopped

DRESSING:

1/2 t. anchovy paste
3 T. olive oil
1/2 t. dried thyme
3 to 5 crushed garlic cloves
2 t. Dijon mustard
3 T. wine vinegar
1 T. dried basil
1 T. parsley
2 T. capers
1 t. fresh ground black pepper
Salt to taste

Mix dressing ingredients together. Place all other ingredients in a large bowl. Pour dressing over and thoroughly mix. Salt to taste. Serve cold.

NOTE: If green beans are frozen, microwave at 30 percent power for 10 minutes stirring at 5 minutes. If you are a tomato lover, add another cup or two of tomatoes.

You can also garnish this salad with left over asparagus, some cucumber slices or raw vegetables.

If you want to make this a "heavier" dish, try serving it with a piece of broiled or barbequed tuna steak and leave the tuna out of the salad.

Potato, Artichoke and Thyme Salad

Serves 4

3 fresh artichokes
2 T. water
1 lb. new potatoes cut into 1 inch chunks
2 T. olive oil
4 cloves (approx. 1/2 T.) minced garlic
1/2 t. dried thyme
Salt and pepper to taste

Place artichokes in a glass pan with water. Cover and microwave artichokes until done (about 15 to 20 minutes). Microwave potatoes on half power for 10 minutes. While the potatoes are cooking, deleaf artichokes and cut hearts into eighths. Saute garlic and thyme in olive oil until garlic browns. Add potatoes and artichoke hearts. Stir until potatoes are slightly browned. Serve warm.

NOTE: You can eat the artichoke leaves as an appetizer with a glass of wine.

Quick Penne Pomodoro (Tube Pasta with Tomatoes)

Serves 4

1 28 oz. can peeled Italian tomatoes
24 oz. penne pasta or rigatoni
4 cloves garlic, sliced
1 t. red pepper flakes
1 t. salt
1 t. dried basil
2 T. olive oil
Shredded Parmesan or romano cheese to garnish

Drain juice from tomatoes and reserve. Cut tomatoes into 1/2 inch pieces. Drain off juice. Cook pasta and drain. While pasta is draining, heat pasta pot to high. Add garlic and pepper.

Saute for 1 minute. Add tomatoes and heat them through. Add pasta back into pot and swirl until pasta is coated. Serve with cheese topping.

Artichoke, Pine Nut Rice Pilaf

Serves 4

1 T. olive oil
1 6 1/2 oz. jar artichoke hearts marinated in olive oil and vinegar
1/3 c. pine nuts
1 t. minced garlic
1 c. small yellow onion, chopped
1 c. rice
2 c. water
1 package dried chicken broth
1 T. lemon juice
Salt and pepper to taste

Drain artichokes and place in sauce pan. Saute artichokes, onion, garlic and pine nuts in olive oil until onion is clear. Add rice and saute 1 minute. Add water, chicken broth package and lemon juice and stir. Bring to a boil then simmer for 20 minutes or until water is absorbed.

NOTE: You can use 2 cups of low salt/low fat chicken broth instead of the water and dried chicken broth if it is available. You can also use Paella type rice to give this recipe a slightly exotic flavor.

Pine Nut Rice Pilaf

Serves 4

1 t. minced garlic
1/4 c. pine nuts
1 large bunch green onions, chopped
2 t. olive oil
1 package chicken broth
2 c. water
1 c. rice

Salt and pepper to taste

Saute pine nuts, onions and garlic in olive oil until nuts and garlic are browned. Add chicken broth and water and rice.

Bring to a boil. Cook for 15 minutes or until water is absorbed by the rice. Serve.

NOTE: You can use 2 cups of low salt/low fat chicken broth instead of the 2 cups of water and packaged chicken broth.

Sicilian Sausage Pasta

Serves 4

2 medium yellow onions, coarsely chopped
1/4 t. anise seeds
1 T. minced garlic
2 T. olive oil
2 fresh bell peppers (yellow, red or green) cored, seeded and cut in 1 inch chunks
1/4 t. crushed red pepper
1/2 lb. turkey Italian sausage, diced
Salt and pepper to taste
1 lb. rotelli or penne or rigatoni pasta
Grated Parmesan or Asiago cheese to taste

Saute onion, anise seeds and garlic in 1 T. olive oil on medium heat until onion is translucent. Add peppers, red pepper flakes, sausage and salt and pepper. Saute until sausage is browned.

Cook pasta until done. Drain pasta and mix with sausage mixture. Add 1 T. olive oil. Stir vigorously over heat approximately 1 minute. Serve with grated cheese topping.

Red Cabbage and Black Bean Soup

Serves 6 to 8

1 head red cabbage
1 piece prosciutto or bacon
1 yellow onion, chopped
2 T. olive oil
4 1/2 quarts water
1 T. minced garlic
1 T. dried oregano
2 t. cumin
Salt and coarsely ground pepper to taste
2 15-oz. cans black beans
1 lb. carrots, chopped
Grated Parmesan cheese to garnish

Core and coarsely chop cabbage. Saute prosciutto and onion in olive oil until onion is translucent. Add cabbage and stir until coated with oil. Add water, spices, beans and carrots. Cook for 1 hour. Serve with grated cheese topping.

Spaghetti Sauce

1 T. olive oil (2 T. if you don't have a non-stick pan)
2 yellow onions, coarsely chopped
1 bell pepper, cored, seeded and coarsely chopped
9 cloves (approx. 1 1/2 T.) garlic, finely minced or crushed
2 4 oz. cans mushrooms, or 8 oz. fresh mushrooms, sliced
1 t. anchovy paste
1 c. red wine
2 T. balsamic vinegar
1 T. Italian spices
1/2 to 1 t. red pepper flakes
1/8 t. anise seed
Salt and pepper to taste
2 large cans (28 oz. each) peeled tomatoes, cut into large pieces, or 3 lbs. fresh Roma tomatoes, peeled and cut into large pieces

Saute onion and peppers in olive oil until onion is translucent. Then add garlic and saute for 1 minute. Turn heat to high and add wine, mushrooms, balsamic vinegar, anchovy paste and spices.

Saute 2 minutes to reduce volume by half. Add tomatoes and bring to near boil. Reduce heat and simmer 2 1/2 to 3 hours.

Summer Squash

Serves 6

3 lbs. yellow crook neck or acorn squash cut into 1 inch chunks
1 T. olive oil
1 large yellow onion coarsely chopped
2 t. minced garlic
1 t. chervil
Parmesan cheese to garnish
Salt and pepper to taste

Microwave squash covered on high for 6 minutes. Saute garlic, chervil and onion in olive oil until onion is translucent, add squash, salt and pepper. Cook over medium low heat for 12 to 15 minutes. Serve with grated cheese over top.

Cumin & Caper Trout

Serves 2

1/2 lb. dressed red meat trout, Coho salmon or snapper
1 T. lemon juice
1 t. minced garlic
1/2 t. ground cumin
1 T. capers (crushed)
1 1/2 T. olive oil
2 T. minced parsley
Salt and pepper to taste
1/2 c. white wine
Arrowroot to thicken sauce

Mix lemon juice, garlic, cumin, capers, 1/2 of olive oil and salt and pepper into a marinade. Marinate fish for at least 15 minutes.

Scrape off marinade before frying. Put the rest of the olive oil in the pan and heat.

Fry in a pan with the marinaded side down for 4 minutes on each side or until the fish is cooked through. Remove fish to a warm plate in oven. Put scraped off marinade and wine into the pan. Reduce by half over a medium high heat.

Turn off heat and add arrowroot to thicken into sauce. Serve sauce over trout. Sprinkle with the rest of of parsley.

NOTE: This recipe can also be made with a microwave by placing the marinaded fish in a glass dish with the marinade, cover and cook for 6 to 8 minutes on high, turning the dish 1/4 turn half way through the cooking. Remove fish and thicken sauce in the microwave using the arrowroot. Pour over fish and garnish with parsley.

Grilled Thyme Tuna (Ahi)

Serves 4

1/4 c. lemon or lime juice
1 lb. tuna steaks, 1 inch thick
2 T. olive oil
1/2 t. dried thyme
1 t. minced garlic
1/4 t. red pepper flakes
1/3 c. white wine
1 8 oz. can mushrooms packed in water, or 1/2 lb. fresh mushrooms, sliced
Salt and pepper to taste

Marinate tuna in lemon juice for 15 minutes. Saute garlic, mushrooms, red pepper flakes and thyme in 1 T. of olive oil at a medium high heat until garlic begins to brown. Add tuna steaks (but not the lemon juice) and cook for 5 minutes on each side. Remove tuna to heated plate. Add wine to pan to deglaze, and reduce stock until only a coating for the mushrooms remains. Serve mushroom mixture over tuna.

Veal Scaloppini

Serves 4

1 lb. thin (1/4 inch thick) boneless veal cutlets
3 T. balsamic vinegar
1/4 t. dried thyme
1/4 t. dried rosemary
1 T. lemon juice
Salt and pepper to taste
4 cloves (approx. 2 t.) minced garlic
2 T. olive oil
Flour to dust cutlets
1/2 c. white wine

Marinate veal in balsamic vinegar, spices, salt and pepper and lemon juice for at least 15 minutes. Saute garlic in olive oil until slightly browned. Lightly dust veal with flour. Add veal and saute over medium heat for 2 minutes on each side. Remove veal from pan and add marinade and wine to pan. Reduce to a light sauce and serve over veal.

Zucchini

Serves 6

2 1/2 lbs. zucchini cut into 1 inch chunks
2 T. olive oil
1 large yellow onion
1/2 T. Italian spices
1/4 t. red pepper flakes
Salt and pepper to taste
1 T. minced garlic
2 T. Balsamic vinegar
Parmesan cheese to garnish

Microwave zucchini covered at half power for 5 minutes. Saute onion, spices and garlic in olive oil at medium high heat until onion is translucent. Add vinegar and zucchini. Cook covered 12 to 15 minutes stirring every 5 minutes. Remove cover and cook until liquid has mostly evaporated. Serve garnished with cheese.

Part V
About The Authors

Keith Ian Marton, M.D.

Chairman of the Department of Medicine, California Pacific Medical Center, Pacific Campus
Clinical Associate Professor, University of California, San Francisco, Medical School

Keith Marton, a general internist, has been the Chairman of the Department of Medicine since 1988. He is also a clinical associ ate professor of medicine at the University of California in San Francisco. A native of Phoenix, Arizona, Dr. Marton received his undergraduate degree in Psychology at Stanford. He graduated from Stanford Medical School in 1970, then completed two years of post-graduate training at Yale-New Haven Hospital in New Haven, Connecticut.

Beginning in 1972, Dr. Marton spent two years as an epidemiologist for the Centers for Disease Control, working primarily at the Los Angeles County Health Department specializing in infectious diseases. In 1974, he returned to Stanford as a senior resident in medicine. He then became chief resident and a fellow in the Robert Wood Johnson Foundation clinical scholars program developing skills in clinical decision making, health economics and health policy issues.

From 1977 until 1984, Dr. Marton was an assistant professor of medicine in the Division of General Medicine at Standard while directing the house-staff teaching program at the Palo Alto VA and serving as that hospital's assistant chief of medicine. In 1984 he established the Division of General Medicine at New England Deaconess Hospital in Boston, administering the department for four years. While in Boston, Dr. Marton was also an associate professor of medicine at Harvard Medical School.

Although he is a general internist in his clinical activities, Marton's research and professional skills are primarily focused in the areas of risk assessment and cost-effective decision making. His research interests are centered on the assessment of heath technology, the psychology of decision making and the cost- effective use of medical resources and have resulted in many articles on decision making in medicine and the co-authoring of a book about clinical decision making.

Wells Shoemaker, M.D.

One Doctor's Journey With Wine and Healing

One of my patients, the intelligent wife of a minister, once asked me how I could dedicate my life to helping children, then turn around and make "alcohol."

I couldn't help but remind her that Jesus performed his first miracle by transforming seven stone cisterns of water into wine. His mother actually urged him to do it, since there was no wine to properly celebrate the wedding in Cana (John 2).

I next blurted out that wine is much more than just alcohol, and in fact, both the medical and the clerical paths have been intertwined with wine through the ages. Wine was part of human civilization long before any of the world's modern religions were organized.

Teenager in Tuscany

I spent six months studying in Florence when I was 19, and it was there that I encountered wine as a matter-of-fact, pleasant, unpretentious part of the evening meal. It wasn't a "score" that I had to make with a fake ID in a liquor store. It wasn't a sexual thrill, and it wasn't a macho overture. It was supper.

I had a Fiat 600 sedan (that's 600 cc engine displacement, smaller than most respectable contemporary motorcycles), and I had a map of Tuscany that had a scale of 1 cm representing 1 km on the ground. I found the roads marked with dotted lines and followed them until they stopped. At the end of each of these roads, I found someone making wine.

Those Tuscan families introduced me to the open, gentle customs of winemaking, to a sense of history in the soil, to a sense of respect among the generations, to sharing with strangers.

I returned to college, and based upon my exposure to the "humanities" in Italy, switched my major from metallurgical engineering to medicine. Some of my medical school classmates were clearly destined for research careers, academic fame, and a few for fortune, but there were a memorable core who took the spirit of the 1960s to their hearts: "Do something real for people." I wanted to be one of them.

I became involved with a farmworkers organization in the San Joaquin Valley and helped to establish a free clinic for migrant workers. While hitchhiking three times a week from Palo Alto to Merced County, I rapidly discovered that the "establishment" shared many of the same health care concerns. I also learned there's no such thing as "free." The free clinic took on a bolder mission.

One of my enduring proud memories was the opening of the Livingston Community Health Center, a clinic owned and serving this entire diverse and energetic community. It recently celebrated its 20th anniversary.

As I churned through medical school and pediatric residency, I also discovered that the world had some wines that far surpassed the ones I could afford. A friend of mine worked at Ridge Vineyards, and he introduced me to the big Ridge Zinfandels of the 1960s. That proved to be a quality standard I've pursued ever since.

Once in private practice in a small rural community, I saw a tremendous pride and energy among people who worked the earth. I also saw a small hospital that had great room--and a certain urgency--to grow in pediatric services. I founded the first intensive care nursery in the Monterey Bay area, and also launched one of the first hospital-based lactation centers in Northern California. In 1985 I published a book on children's medications entitled *Little Ills and Bitter Pills.*

I also could finally afford bottles with corks. After a few years of visiting wineries and learning how to taste wine, I wanted to do it myself. I guess I'd rather be a wine player than a wine Spectator.

Starting as a home winemaker, with some timely guidance from Jeff Baker (now winemaker at Carmenet), I rapidly began to appreciate the challenge of doing it right. For about ten years, I took as many courses in winemaking at University of California, Davis Extension courses and Napa Valley centers as I did in continuing pediatric education.

The home wines did very well in competitions, but the quest for better quality grapes, new French oak barrels, and better tools began to consume a great deal of time and money. It wasn't a hobby any more. I received a great deal of encouragement, and with a gulp, I opened Salamandre Wine Cellars as a commercial, bonded winery in 1985.

The grape harvest has put smiles on people's faces and aches in people's backs since the pre-history of the Mediterranean. At the end of the day in October, I'll be sitting on a stack of dirty lug boxes, hairs all stuck together with must, T shirt stiff and dirty, grinning like a kid at some large circular container full of crushed purple grapes. At the same time, some guy and his wife are sitting on a stack of boxes in Portugal and Italy and France and Greece and Russia with the same grin. In wine there is a unity among people that transcends politics and language, and it goes back in time long before even democracy was invented.

Wine and Health

In the early 1980s, I began collecting medical information about wine, and I was amused that there was actually a legitimate body of science on the subject. It made entertaining coffee-table conversation.

The politicization of alcohol issues, using health claims as a central focus, removed wine and health from the coffee table and thrust it into the media battlefield. I became first annoyed ... and then outraged by the self-righteous distortion of balance by national agencies charged with public health.

I dug into the scientific literature in earnest. I've written for several trade journals, and serve as chairman of the Scientific Advisory Board to the Wine Institute of California.

Conflict of Interest

I've been amused by comments I overhear when I talk to medical and winemaking audiences. The winemakers seem to say, "Here's another dilettante doctor tax-dodger getting into the wine business. "The doctors say politely, "Well, how can you be objective since you're making all that money in the wine business?"

To winemakers, I say that Salamandre Wine Cellars produces about 2,000 cases of wine a year; you might say Tuscan hillside dimensions. That comes from around 30 tons of grapes, practically all of which I've personally lifted three or four times before turning it into juice I can pump. Two thousand cases is a tiny amount compared to most Napa Valley wineries, and a mere speck of mist in the eyes of the very largest. But that 2,000 cases of product weighs 40 tons, and that's a lot of boxes to shuffle without a fork-lift.

For the doctors, I have to remind them that I didn't choose pediatrics for its investment potential. If small winery economics were ever to distort my objectivity, it would probably be to provoke a woozy headshake about my financial foolhardiness.

After seven years of a backbreaking, sweaty, gritty labor of love, Salamandre finally broke even in 1991. Maybe the winery will eventually subsidize the college educations of my daughters. Hardly the sort of money that makes a man sell out his scruples. Personally, I'm holding out for a lot more money before I let anybody get their hands on my scruples.

Science speaks clearly and I gain nothing by twisting it. Jiminy Cricket told Pinochio, "When in doubt, tell the truth." That's good advice; I wish the government would try it.

Lewis Perdue
Author:
Almost Scientist, Accidental Journalist

Lewis Perdue almost became a scientist, but wound up a journalist instead -- mostly by accident and economic necessity.

Perdue started his college education in electrical engineering, working in the summers as a technician for Westinghouse Electric where he worked on a variety of projects including building instrumentation for space satellites, calibrating instruments used in nuclear reactors and wiring circuits used in lab equipment.

He gradually changed his interest to physics and then biophysics. As a biology/physics major at Cornell University, Perdue supported himself financially by working as a reporter for the local Gannett chain newspaper, *The Ithaca Journal*, and by selling freelance magazine articles.

Perdue had earlier gotten an A.S. degree in math and science from Corning College (becoming the first student in the college's history to graduate with a perfect 4.0 grade point average) while working as a reporter for another Gannett newspaper, *The Elmira Star-Gazette.*

By the end of his junior year at Cornell (and lacking only three courses for his major) Perdue decided that being a journalist was more rewarding than being a scientist. While it took a number of special petitions to academic committees, he was eventually allowed to convert his science courses into electives and take all of his major subjects in the two semesters of his senior year. He graduated first in his major with a B.S. in Communications in 1972.

Since then, Perdue has worked as a Washington correspondent, investigative reporter, business journalist, Congressional news secretary, computer marketing consultant and computer industry reporter. Along the way, he also managed to write 13 books in addition to this one.

Following his graduation from Cornell, Perdue worked full-time for the *Ithaca Journal*, taught magazine writing at Cornell and then took a job with Mississippi Gov. Bill Waller. Waller was famous for his earlier work as the district attorney who prosecuted the assassin of civil rights advocate Medgar Evers despite death threats and pressure from the state's segregationist-controlled Democratic Party.

Earlier, in 1967, Perdue was kicked out of the University of Mississippi for leading a demonstration. The incident was somewhat embarrassing for the family since Perdue's great- grandfather had once been chancellor at Ole Miss; his grandfather had been a chemistry professor there and his father worked for the governor at the time. An even earlier relative, great-great- grandfather James Z. George was a U.S. Senator, chief justice of the state Supreme Court, author of the state's post-Civil-War constitution and the creator of Jim Crow

Segregation -- embodying in the constitution the literacy test and the poll tax.

Four years after being expelled from Ole Miss, Perdue wrote a seminal (and widely reprinted) piece on "The New South" for *The Nation*, theorizing why he and some others of his generation had rejected the racist culture that had nurtured them.

The work for Waller thrust Perdue into the public eye and into a hotbed of political intrigue. Perdue later went to Washington D.C. to work as news secretary to moderate Congressman Thad Cochran, and later to help manage and consult for campaigns for liberal Republican candidates for Congress, a task he describes as "more frustrating than waiting for Godot."

Frustrated with politics, Perdue returned to journalism. His most prominent investigative reporting experience came in 1977 when, as a freelance journalist, he helped break the Koreagate Congressional bribery scandal. During that time, his freelance articles were printed in *The Washington Post, Jack Anderson's column, Washington Monthly,* and wrote a weekly column for the Washington bureau of Gannett News Service.

In addition to his work on Koreagate, Perdue wrote the first articles on Congressional misuse of perks, sex discrimination on Congressional staffs and even about an illegal gambling ring for Congressmen and their staffs which operated with the knowledge of the Capitol Police Force.

Following his freelance work, Perdue served as a correspondent covering the White House, Congress and Supreme Court for Dow Jones/Ottaway Newspapers and for States News Service.

It was as a reporter in the nation's capital that Perdue realized that members of the U.S. government has institutionalized the act of lying to each other and to country's citizens. Like parts of this book, many of Perdue's articles documented the ways that bureaucrats and public officials lie to protect their turf and to advance the hidden agendas that frequently diverged from the public interest.

Of particular interest to him was the ways in which government distorted and misused scientific data. His scientific education gave him the background -- unusual among journalists -- to understand when and how data were being twisted for ulterior motives.

Finally, in early 1979 -- disgusted beyond tolerance for politics -- Perdue went to Los Angeles where he taught journalism at UCLA and also served as advisor to the student daily newspaper there. During this time, he served as the editorial page editor of the *Santa Monica Evening Outlook* where his work was nominated for a Pulitzer Prize.

Already the author of two books by this time, Perdue began writing in earnest with two bestsellers (*The Delphi Betrayal, 1981* and *Queensgate Reckoning, 1982, Pinnacle Books.*)

He also continued his freelance work, writing for *The Los Angeles Times, California Magazine, California Business Magazine* and others. His life took an abrupt turn in 1984 when UCLA abolished the journalism department because the university administration felt it was too "trade-school like" and not sufficiently academic. On the heels of this setback, the publisher of Perdue's bestsellers went bankrupt in 1984 (still owing Perdue most of his royalties). Perdue quickly put his technical and writing education to work for several firms which provided marketing and public relations services to computer firms.

Perdue eventually started his own consulting firm, sold it in 1990 and moved to Sonoma, Calif. in the fall of 1990.

Along the way, Perdue found time to conduct technical product reviews and write for *PC World, InfoWorld, Publish!, Computer Currents* and other computer magazines. He also wrote the first book on how to upgrade IBM PCs.

In February 1991, he founded *Wine Business Insider* a fortnightly newsletter covering the management, finance, regulatory, marketing and other business aspects of the wine industry. *Wine Business Insider* is now the largest circulation trade newsletter in the American wine industry.

In addition to the *Insider,* Perdue regularly writes for the *San Francisco Chronicle*

♥